Contraception in Practice

Edited by

Stephen Killick, MD, FRCOG

Professor and Head, Department of
Obstetrics and Gynaecology
University of Hull
Director, Hull IVF Unit, UK

MARTIN DUNITZ

© Martin Dunitz Ltd 2000

First published in the United Kingdom in 2000
by Martin Dunitz Ltd, The Livery House, 7–9 Pratt Street, London NW1 0AE

A CIP record for this book is available from the British Library.

ISBN 1 85317 791 1

Distributed in the USA, Canada and Brazil by Blackwell Science Inc., Commerce Place, 250 Main Street, Malden, MA 02148–5018, USA
Tel. 1–800–215–1000

Composition by Wearset, Boldon, Tyne and Wear
Printed and bound in Italy by Printer Trento

Contents

List of contributors

Alison Bigrigg
Glasgow Centre for Family Planning and Reproductive Health
6 Sandyford Place
Sauciehall Street
Glasgow G3 7NB, UK

Urszula Bankowska
Glasgow Centre for Family Planning and Reproductive Health
6 Sandyford Place
Sauciehall Street
Glasgow G3 7NB, UK

Elaine Cooper
Learning Disability Team
Community Health Services NHS Trust
Hawthorn Lodge
Moorgreen Hospital
Southampton SO30 3JB, UK

Linda Egdell
Family Planning Service
Royal Alexandra Hospital
Marine Drive
Rhyl, Denbighshire LL18 3AS, UK

Ailsa Gebbie
Family Planning and Well Woman Services
18 Dean Terrace
Edinburgh EH4 1NL, UK

Babatunde A Gbolade
Fertility Control Unit
St James's University Hospital
Beckett Street
Leeds LS9 7TF, UK

Anna Glasier
Family Planning and Well Woman Services
18 Dean Terrace
Edinburgh EH4 1NL, UK

David Hicks
Department of Genito-Urinary Medicine
Royal Hallamshire Hospital
Glossop Road
Sheffield S10 2JF, UK

Stephen Killick
Department of Obstetrics and Gynaecology
University of Hull
Princess Royal Hospital
Saltshouse Road
Hull HU8 9HE, UK

Anne MacGregor
City of London Migraine Clinic
22 Charterhouse Square
London EC1M 6DX, UK

Kay McAllister
Glasgow Centre for Family Planning and
Reproductive Health
6 Sandyford Place
Sauciehall Street
Glasgow G3 7NB, UK

Michael O'Connell
Dept of Obstetrics and Gynaecology
University of Hull
Princess Royal Hospital
Saltshouse Road
Hull HU8 9HE, UK

Nicholas Panay
Fertility Centre
St Bartholomew's Hospital
West Smithfield
London EC1A 7BE, UK

Botros Rizk
Department of Obstetrics and Gynaecology
University of South Alabama College of
Medicine
Suite 100, 251 Cox Street
Mobile, AL 36604, USA

Anne Szarewski
Imperial Cancer Research Fund
PO Box 123
Lincoln's Inn Fields
London WC2A 3PX, UK

Ian H Thorneycroft
Department of Obstetrics and Gynaecology
University of South Alabama College of
Medicine
Suite 100, 251 Cox Street
Mobile, AL 36604, USA

Kate Weaver
Family Planning and Well Woman Services
18 Dean Terrace
Edinburgh EH4 1NL, UK

Introduction

Family planning is often considered in isolation from general medicine. This is particularly true in the UK, with many family planning clinics functioning separately from general practice surgeries, but it is true to some extent in all parts of the world. The reason for this is, of course, that most patients who request contraceptive advice are otherwise completely healthy.

A good example of this isolated approach is the way family planning is taught. We learn the failure rates, complications and relative costs of each contraceptive method such as oral contraception, IUCDs and Norplant rather than considering the needs of patients like Janet, who may have breast cancer, or John, who may be oligospermic. It may be acceptable to consider contraceptive provision to otherwise completely healthy women in this way but an increasing number of requests for contraception come from individuals who have a pre-existing medical problem. Dealing effectively with these family planning problems demands a far wider expertise than merely knowledge of contraceptive methods.

This textbook looks at the subject from a different angle. Medical conditions that occur commonly in women of reproductive age are described in some detail and then the factors that might affect the choice of contraceptive in each particular case are discussed. It should be no surprise that contraception is an integral part of the clinical management of many young women with minor or sometimes serious medical conditions. In many cases it is the non-contraceptive action of hormonal contraceptives that provides the benefit.

Examples in this book range from polycystic ovaries to breast cancer. Chapters also deal with non-medical conditions such as the particular problems encountered by teenagers or couples with learning difficulties. This means that the chapters differ greatly in their style, some being primarily discussions of pathophysiology, while others concentrate on the more social aspects. All the authors,

however, have emphasized the practical aspects of treating patients and each chapter concludes with short case histories in order to illustrate the points raised. I am sure you will identify your own patients in these case histories, including the final discussion of patients for whom no form of contraception seems to be suitable.

It is always the case that the best advice is obtained from those with the greatest experience but that these individuals have the least free time to commit their experiences to paper. All the authors who have contributed to this book are working day in, day out, with the type of patients they describe. I am extremely grateful for their time and willingness to write about contraception from this slightly different point of view.

Stephen Killick

Women with breast cancer

Kate Weaver and Anna Glasier

1

Breast cancer is the most common malignancy among women and the UK has the highest incidence and mortality associated with this disease worldwide. It is estimated that 1 in 12 British women develops breast cancer at some time in her life. The age-specific incidence of breast cancer is such that many women are affected at a relatively young age, compared with other cancers. Five-year survival rates after treatment of early stage tumours can be up to 90%, but the risk of survivors developing cancer in the contralateral breast is 1% per year.

One in 12 British women develops breast cancer at some time in her life

These statistics explain why there are many premenopausal breast cancer survivors who need good advice about contraceptives that will not increase their chances of recurrent breast cancer. Some women will wish to conceive and want to know the impact this might have on their future risk of breast cancer, and many women wonder if hormone replacement therapy (HRT) will be safe for them. Women may seek advice and support if they experience disruption of their sexual activity after treatment of breast cancer, but are often reticent about mentioning problems of this nature.

There is an even larger group of young women with a family history of breast cancer. These women have an increased risk of breast cancer and with much or all of their reproductive careers ahead of them, need to know how pregnancy and contraceptives may affect that risk. Those with a particularly strong family history may be at higher risk and the question of genetic screening arises.

This chapter addresses these concerns, which are better understood in light of the probable relationship between breast cancer and female hormones, briefly discussed below.

Relationship between breast cancer and hormones

Endogenous hormones

There is much evidence to suggest that both exogenous and endogenous hormones have a role in the aetiology of breast cancer. Established risk factors include early menarche, late menopause, nulliparity and late age at first full-term pregnancy. Each of these factors is associated with a doubling or tripling of breast cancer risk, and each is linked with prolonged

exposure to endogenous oestrogens and progesterone. Bone mineral density is a marker of lifetime exposure to oestrogen and in one US study of older women, bone mineral density was positively correlated with risk of breast cancer (Cauley et al. 1996). It is thought that this hormone exposure acts indirectly, by generating an increased population of the undifferentiated epithelial stem cells in the breast which are susceptible to the initial stages in cell transformation towards fully malignant cells (Thomas 1984).

High, unopposed endogenous oestrogen levels also seem to be a factor in the pathogenesis of some breast cancers. Groups of women with late menopause, obesity, polycystic ovary syndrome and oestrogen-secreting tumours all have increased incidence of breast cancer.

Exogenous hormones

There is much debate about the role of hormonal contraception and HRT in the aetiology of breast cancer. Results from a collaborative reanalysis of virtually all the data available worldwide from studies of breast cancer and hormonal contraceptives (Collaborative Group on Hormonal Factors in Breast Cancer 1996) show a 24% higher rate of breast cancer in women while taking combined oral contraceptives, compared with women who have never taken oral contraceptives (relative risk 1.24; confidence interval 1.15 to 1.33) The increased risk persists after women stop taking oral contraceptives but steadily declines so that there is no excess of cancers 10 or more years after stopping use. It appears that breast cancers in women who have used oral contraceptives are likely to be clinically less advanced at diagnosis, with a better prognosis than cancers in women who have never used oral contraceptives. The magnitude of increased risk varies across age groups. Ongoing oral contraceptive use beginning before the age of 20 years seems to carry an almost 60% increased risk (RR 1.59 ± 0.93). However, this is not statistically significant, and clinically it applies at an age when breast cancer incidence is low, so that it represents a very small number of actual cases (*Figure 1*).

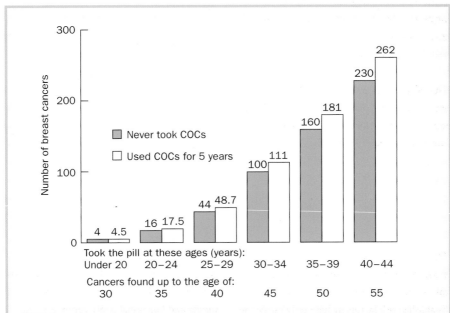

Figure 1
Excess breast cancers associated with 5 years of COC use. Estimated cumulative numbers of breast cancers per 10 000 women diagnosed in 5 years of use and up to 10 years after stopping COCs, compared with numbers of breast cancers diagnosed in 10 000 women who never used COCs. Reproduced with permission from Current Problems in Pharmacovigilance *(1998)* **24**: *2–3.*

No dose relationship was demonstrable and neither duration of use nor type of hormone had any significant impact on risk.

There is a 24% higher rate of breast cancer in women who are taking oral contraceptives

Progestogen-only methods were less well represented in the studies reanalysed. However, the results suggest a similar association; the rate of breast cancer was up by 17% (relative risk 1.17) for use of oral progestogen-only methods within the previous 5 years, compared with non-users. Users of injectable progestogens also had a 17% increased risk of breast cancer, but this was not statistically significant (relative risk 1.17). No increased risk was found in women who had stopped these methods 10 or more years before.

Possible mechanisms of pathogenesis

These findings could be explained by earlier detection of breast cancer in users of hormonal contraception, particularly as both combined and progestogen-only methods share the same pattern of increase in cancers diagnosed during use and 5–10 years thereafter. Alternatively, there may be a causal link, in late stage promotion of tumours. This would be compatible with the excess of early stage tumours diagnosed up to 10 years after cessation of hormonal contraception. The apparent connection between hormonal contraception and breast cancer could be the result of a combination of biological factors and better detection.

Evidence from HRT use

Hormone replacement therapy is also associated with an increased risk of breast cancer. In contrast with the findings on hormonal contraceptives, there is evidence of a dose- and duration-dependent effect, suggesting a causal relationship. Less than 5 years of HRT is not consistently associated with increased risk, but 5 or more years of use increases the risk of breast cancer by around 50% for women in their fifties and around 70% for those in their sixties (Colditz et al. 1995). In one study, 0.625 mg per day of conjugated oestrogens had no effect but 1.25 mg per day was associated with a doubling of risk (Dupont and Page 1991). Oestrogen-only and combined preparations appear to have the same impact on risk. As with oral contraceptives, the breast cancers diagnosed during and shortly after HRT use are generally lower-grade tumours with a better prognosis than those in never-users of HRT (Harding et al. 1996).

Hormone replacement therapy of less than 5 years' duration does not increase the risk of breast cancer

Clinical implications

The huge volume of literature on the relationship between exogenous hormones and breast cancer is valuable both in understanding the aetiology of the disease and in counselling women on contraceptive and HRT choices. Breast cancer is only weakly related to hormonal milieu, and other significant factors such as genetics and diet must be at play. Nevertheless, breast cancer is common, it is widely feared and has been linked with contraception and HRT in the popular press, so the issue is often raised by patients in consultations about HRT or contraception. For most women, the data are reassuring. Any increase in breast cancer risk associated with the combined oral contraceptive (COC) is balanced against protection from endometrial and ovarian cancers and the undoubted benefits of reliable protection from unwanted pregnancy. All reproductive decisions involve such factors in a complicated risk–benefit analysis. The majority of women appreciate the facts being put to them clearly, and are prepared then to make their own choices.

It is harder to advise women in high-risk groups. Those who have already suffered from breast cancer have a high recurrence risk; after wide local excision and radiotherapy, recurrence rate in the treated breast is 1% per year. There is also a higher chance of developing a tumour in the contralateral breast. Women with a family history can have a breast cancer risk double that of the general population. For women from high-risk families with a 'cancer gene' there is an approximately 85% lifetime risk of developing the disease (Dixon 1995). The following sections deal with these special groups.

Reproductive decisions after breast cancer

Contraception

Many women will be rendered infertile by the systemic treatment of their breast malignancy, either permanently or temporarily. Ovarian ablation (surgical or radiation) is less often performed now but clearly leads to permanent infertility and there will be no further need for contraception. Tamoxifen suppresses ovulation in some patients but is not reliably contraceptive and barrier contraception is recommended during its use, particularly in view of concerns about pregnancy complications in women taking this drug. After discontinuing tamoxifen, ovulation may resume if it had been suppressed, although many older women may develop

MEDICAL ELIGIBILITY CRITERIA FOR THE USE OF CONTRACEPTIVES (WHO 1996)

Category	Description
1	A condition for which there is no restriction for the use of the contraceptive method. The method can be used with limited clinical judgement
2	A condition in which the advantages of using the method generally outweigh the theoretical or proven risks. The method can be used with limited clinical judgement
3	A condition in which the theoretical or proven risks generally outweigh the advantages of using the method and it should only be used as method of last choice, when other methods are unavailable or unacceptable. Clinical judgement is required and patients should be followed up carefully
4	A condition in which the contraceptive method represents an unacceptable health risk. The method should not be used under any circumstances

permanent amenorrhoea (Surbone and Petrek 1997). Multiple-agent chemotherapy causes medical menopause and permanent infertility in varying numbers of women, depending on the dose and type of chemotherapy and the age of the patient. For example, one study looked at women under 35 years old on doxorubicin: 59% continued to menstruate, 32% were temporarily amenorrhoeic and 9% were persistently amenorrhoeic. After therapy with cyclophosphamide, melphalan and fluorouracil, younger women are unlikely to become permanently amenorrhoeic, but the chances of this increase dramatically after the age of 35 years (Surbone and Petrek 1997).

Clearly, there will be many premenopausal women who become amenorrhoeic during systemic therapy, a significant proportion of whom will subsequently regain fertility, especially among the under-35 age group. It seems advisable for all these women to assume they are potentially fertile and require contraception until they have been well, off treatment, and amenorrhoeic for 2 years.

Contraceptive options

In its guidelines on quality care in family planning, the World Health Organization assigns medical eligibility criteria from 1 to 4 for the use of contraceptives in different medical conditions (WHO 1996). These replace the concept of relative and absolute contraindications, aiming to optimize choice within acceptable margins of safety. The criteria are broad and simple, and designed to serve as a starting point for the development of relevant national guidelines in diverse circumstances (see box on page 6).

Combined oral contraceptive pills

The body of evidence linking oestrogens and progestogens with breast cancer is strong enough to deter the majority of doctors, and women themselves, from ever using hormonal contraceptives after a diagnosis of breast cancer. There is a wide choice of alternative, safe contraceptive methods.

The World Health Organization's medical eligibility criteria suggest that COCs should not be used at all in women with current breast cancer (category 4). In those who are free of disease 5 years after treatment for breast cancer, COCs should only be used with clinical judgement when more suitable options are not applicable (category 3). Applying these guidelines in the context of the developed world, it is reasonable for women in this latter group to use the COC if they stand to gain from its health benefits, are well informed of the potential risks and are prepared to be closely monitored.

Injectable combined contraceptives are not yet available in the UK, but are widely used in South America. Combined oestrogen–progestogen patch and vaginal ring products

are both in development in the UK. The same considerations will apply to these contraceptives as they come into general use.

Progestogen-only methods

The reanalysis of global data on oral contraceptives (Collaborative Group on Hormonal Factors in Breast Cancer 1996) had more limited information on progestogen-only methods, because these methods have been less widely used than combined oral contraceptives. As with COCs, there seems to be a small elevation of risk during use, and for several years after discontinuing use.

The injectable contraceptive depot medroxyprogesterone acetate (DMPA) has been linked with breast cancer since early in its development when beagle dogs suffered a high incidence of mammary tumours. This hampered licensing of DMPA as a contraceptive in the USA until 1992. Even in the many countries where it is widely and successfully used, ill-founded concerns persist. The beagle is now discredited as a useful model for steroid administration in humans. More importantly, large studies have shown that DMPA is associated with only a marginally increased rate of breast cancer in women, possibly owing to increased detection rather than a causal relationship with the disease.

The WHO medical eligibility criteria guidelines are broadly similar to those for COCs, but are more conservative about injections and implants. This probably reflects the relative lack of data rather than any biological basis for concern. Injections and implants are category 4 in current breast cancer. The progestogen-only pill and the levonorgestrel intrauterine system (IUS) should be discontinued if in use at the time of diagnosis (category 4) but may be initiated *de novo* if no other method is possible in a woman with current breast cancer (category 3). After 5 years of disease-free survival, women may use any progestogen-only method as a last resort, if non-hormonal methods are not suitable (category 3). The medical eligibility criteria are summarized in *Table 1*.

The levonorgestrel-releasing IUS has theoretical benefits of reducing the risk of endometrial hyperplasia in women on tamoxifen and hence reducing endometrial cancer risk, without significant systemic absorption of levonorgestrel. Studies of this effect are in progress.

Barrier methods

Non-hormonal contraceptives cannot have any impact on breast cancer risk and the WHO guidelines put no restriction on their use. Women who are amenorrhoeic during and after systemic therapy may wish to use these methods while waiting to see if they are permanently amenorrhoeic. Vaginal dryness can make condoms uncomfortable to use and the diaphragm less easy for women to fit. Simple

Table 1
The WHO medical eligibility criteria for contraceptive use in breast disease.

Condition	Category				
	COC	POP	DMPA/NET-EN	NOR	LNG IUS
Family history of breast cancer	1	1	1	1	1
Past breast cancer, no evidence of current disease for 5 years	3	3	3	3	3
Current breast cancer:					
Initiation of method	4	3	4	4	3
Continuation of method	4	4	4	4	4
Benign breast disease	1	1	1	1	1

COC, combined oral contraceptive; POP, progestogen-only pill; DMPA, depot medroxyprogesterone acetate; NET-EN, norethisterone enanthanate; NOR, Norplant; LNG IUS, levonorgestrel intrauterine system.

lubricants and spermicidal gels help, but oestrogen creams should generally be avoided in women with current or recent breast cancer because of fears about systemic absorption.

Intrauterine devices

There is no reason to limit the use of non-medicated intrauterine devices.

Sterlization (male or female)

A reliable, permanent method of non-hormonal birth control is attractive. The irreversible nature of sterilization means that it is unwise to make hasty decisions at a time of crisis around a diagnosis of cancer.

Pregnancy

Ovulation is suppressed in some but not all patients taking continuous tamoxifen. Many women will be rendered permanently infertile by their adjuvant cancer therapy. These women may in future be helped by ovarian autotransplantation. The technology currently exists for harvesting and cryopreserving ovarian tissue, and thawing viable oocytes. It is not yet possible, however, to mature human oocytes in vitro (Oehninger 1998).

For women who retain fertility and wish to consider pregnancy, the data are broadly reassuring. Several large studies of pregnancy after breast cancer have found that neither full-term nor aborted pregnancies have any impact on breast cancer survival (Kroman et al. 1997). These findings, however, are based on well women, with a good outcome from breast cancer treatment, since sicker women will be more likely to lose fertility or to be advised against pregnancy.

The UK Royal College of Obstetricians and Gynaecologists issued guidelines on this subject in 1997. They recommended that women wait 2–3 years after treatment, by which time disease-free survival is a reasonable indicator of long-term survival (RCOG 1997). Women planning a pregnancy are advised to consult their oncologist, surgeon and an obstetrician beforehand. Those who become pregnant after breast cancer should be managed by this team in close consultation. Women who inadvertently become pregnant can make their decision about continuing or terminating the pregnancy in the knowledge that neither option is likely to worsen or improve their prognosis. Prior breast cancer treatment does not appear to affect the health of the offspring (Myers and Schilsky 1992), although there are concerns about pregnancies conceived in women taking tamoxifen.

Hormone replacement therapy

After natural or induced menopause, breast cancer survivors may seek relief of menopausal symptoms. Small studies of HRT in breast cancer survivors have not demonstrated any increased risk of recurrence (DiSaia et al. 1995). Only well women are likely to enrol in such studies, so their findings need to be interpreted with caution. Women taking HRT at the time of primary breast cancer diagnosis have a better prognosis than others (Harding et al. 1996). A previous history of breast cancer remains a contraindication on the data sheets of all HRT preparations. Official guidelines such as those from the Scottish Intercollegiate Guidelines Network (1998) advise non-oestrogen alternatives such as megestrol acetate, progestogens and soya proteins. When these preparations fail to alleviate severe menopausal symptoms, there is a growing feeling that HRT may justifiably be prescribed, after careful counselling (Braendle 1998). Larger studies addressing this question are in progress.

Women with a family history of breast cancer

The diagnosis of breast cancer in a close relative is not only devastating for the family but also raises the spectre of increased personal breast cancer risk. Women may want to know how likely it is that they too will develop breast cancer and whether it is still safe for them to use hormonal contraceptives or HRT.

The current literature on the heritability of breast cancer can be bewildering, perhaps because there remain large areas of uncertainty, in a field which is still research-dominated, but is being put into clinical practice in screening programmes before the full clinical implications are known.

A family history of breast cancer elevates risk to around twice that of the general population; however, there are some families whose members are at considerably higher risk and for whom referral to specialist clinics may be advisable. The following section deals first with these women and then with women whose family pedigree does not merit specialist referral.

High-risk families

The following categories of women are at substantially increased risk of breast cancer (three or more times that of the general population) and should be considered for referral to specialist clinics (Scottish Collegiate Guidelines Network 1998):

- one first-degree relative with bilateral breast cancer or breast plus ovarian cancer, *or*

- one first-degree relative with breast cancer diagnosed before age 40 years or one first-degree male relative with breast cancer at any age, *or*

- two first- or second-degree relatives with breast cancer under age 60 years, or ovarian cancer at any age, on the same side of the family, *or*

- three first- or second-degree relatives with breast or ovarian cancer on the same side of the family.

Women at very high risk in whom direct gene testing may be appropriate include those with four or more relatives affected with breast or ovarian cancer in three generations and one living affected individual.

High-risk families—also characterized as carrying 'hereditary breast cancer syndromes'—are those whose family pedigree suggests the presence of a single gene autosomal dominant mutation with high penetrance, causing breast (and often other) cancers, usually at a younger age than in the general population. Numerous mutations have now been characterized in the *BRCA1* and *BRCA2* genes. Mutations in *BRCA1* are associated also with a high incidence of ovarian cancer in women and of prostate and colon cancers in male members of the families. Mutations in *BRCA2* are less strongly associated with ovarian cancer, but are linked to other epithelial malignancies, of larynx, prostate and pancreas, as well as male breast cancer.

Estimates vary as to what proportion of high-risk families carry mutations in one of these genes. The early suggestion that 50% of such families carried *BRCA1* mutations now seems to have been an overestimate. Recent studies have found incidences as low as 12.8% in some high-risk clinic populations. On the other hand, it is acknowledged that these long genes probably harbour many yet-uncharacterized mutations. The population incidence of *BRCA1* mutation has been estimated at 1 in 500 to 1 in 1000, but certain groups, such as Ashkenazi Jews, have a substantially higher incidence (Couch and Hartmann 1998).

Other rare heritable cancer syndromes such as ataxia telangiectasia account for a further small subgroup of heritable breast cancers.

Occasionally, women with a weak (or no) family history of breast cancer can carry mutations in *BRCA1*, *BRCA2* or other 'cancer' genes. Small families may not manifest a hereditary breast cancer syndrome as dramatically as larger families, and this is a factor taken into account when specialists construct family pedigrees.

Screening should certainly be carried out in specialist clinics with full counselling about the clinical, psychological, employment and insurance consequences of screening, whatever the result. It is also important that women understand the current imperfect state of the screening tests and accept that a negative result at best leaves them with the normal background population risk of breast cancer, and at worst may mean that an unknown mutation has been missed. In this connection, it is helpful to be able to test family members who have developed the disease, so that any mutation detected can then be specifically sought in their relatives. Screening should be carried out in the context of research programmes so that knowledge can advance. In this specialist setting, women who do have genetic mutations predisposing to breast (and other) cancers may be offered regular screening, tamoxifen prophylaxis (in the setting of ongoing clinical trials) or even prophylactic mastectomies and oophorectomies. None of these strategies is guaranteed to prevent malignancies arising and careful specialist advice and counselling are essential.

Recommendations regarding contraception, HRT and pregnancy in this very high-risk group should come from specialists. Recent work suggests that the COC reduces the risk of ovarian cancer significantly in carriers of *BRCA1/2* mutations (Narod et al. 1998). These women are probably more at risk of breast cancer on the COC (Ursin et al. 1997), but this is more easily screened for and treated than ovarian cancer. This trade-off may be justified and specialists could in future be advocating COC use as prophylaxis for this group of patients.

Other women with a family history of breast cancer

It is important to remember that only 5–10% of UK breast cancers have a known genetic element and that the majority of women with a family history of breast cancer do not have a defined breast cancer syndrome. The occurrence of more than one case of breast cancer in a given family might be explained by simple coincidence (breast cancer is a common malignancy), common environmental exposures, or perhaps recessive or variably penetrant genetic traits as yet undiscovered. Women with more than one case of breast cancer in the family have, however, twice the general population incidence of breast cancer. Current thinking is that specialist referral is not merited, but these women may nonetheless want to know how hormonal contraceptives might affect their risk of developing breast cancer.

Combined oral contraceptive pill

Studies of the interaction of family history and COC use have given conflicting conclusions (Murray et al. 1989, Calle et al. 1993). The 1996 collaborative reanalysis of data on breast cancer and oral contraceptives included the available data on possible interactions. The small increase in breast cancer incidence associated with current or recent oral contraceptive use is no higher in women with a family history of breast cancer than in those without. However, this comparison is based on small numbers of women and should be interpreted with caution.

A large review of the epidemiological literature (Thomas 1991) concluded that COCs do not appear to potentiate the effects of other risk factors. Nine of the studies reviewed looked at the relative risk of breast cancer, in women with and without a family history, on the COC. Women with a family history did not have higher relative risk of breast cancer in any study. More broadly, Thomas found no evidence that any known high-risk group had further increased risk on the COC. He suggests that those at high risk may already have maximal stimulation of the breast cancer cell populations susceptible to malignant change, so that they cannot respond to any further stimulation from exogenous hormones.

A family history of breast cancer is not relevant for women using combined oral contraception

On the basis of the above work, WHO guidelines state that a family history of breast cancer is not relevant for women using the COC, and that it can be used without

limitation in this group (WHO 1996). They do not make any distinction between women with a very high-risk family history of breast cancer and those with perhaps just one relative who developed breast cancer later in life.

Progestogen-only methods

Again, the data are limited and the WHO guidelines place no restriction on any progestogen-only method in these women. If the reliability and convenience of hormonal contraception is required, with minimal hormonal dose, the levonorgestrel IUS may be a good option.

Non-hormonal methods

No restrictions are placed on any non-hormonal methods by the WHO guidelines in women with a family history of breast cancer.

Pregnancy

The changes in relative risk of breast cancer associated with pregnancy or nulliparity are too small to figure in personal family planning decisions. A simple family history of breast cancer need not be a contraindication to pregnancy.

Hormone replacement therapy

If an individual woman has inherited a

predisposition to breast cancer, this will usually have manifested itself within 5 years of the age at which her relative was diagnosed. The strength of the association between family history and personal risk of breast cancer mortality decreases with age and after passing through the menopause (Calle et al. 1993), so for menopausal women the fear of inheriting a familial breast cancer tendency is beginning to abate.

As with COCs, the risk factors of family history and HRT do not seem to interact. In meta-analysis of 10 studies, women with a family history of breast cancer did not have increased rates of breast cancer on HRT compared with those with no family history (Colditz et al. 1993). The finding of lower breast cancer mortality in women on HRT at time of diagnosis is also reassuring (Harding et al. 1996).

Sexual relations after breast cancer diagnosis and treatment

Between 21% and 39% of women report long-term sexual problems after breast cancer treatment, either ceasing to enjoy sex or no longer having intercourse (Anderson 1985, Weijmar et al. 1995). This is significant because sex is an aspect of a loving, supportive relationship which can aid women's emotional and thereby physical well-being after breast cancer (Spiegel et al. 1989).

Between 21% and 39% of women report long-term sexual problems after breast cancer treatment

A number of problems can conspire to cause sexual dissatisfaction for couples after diagnosis and treatment of breast cancer. It is easy to understand that physical problems such as postoperative pain, hypersensitivity after radiotherapy and the consequences of abrupt medical menopause can all affect libido and sexual function. However, studies consistently show that psychological factors are much more important determinants of sexual outcome. Distorted body image damages feelings of attractiveness. Anxiety and depression interfere with libido and arousal. There may also be specific fears about sex affecting the prognosis, or causing cancer in the other breast. Aspects of the relationship may be problematic, or helpful. Couples with a supportive, loving relationship and a good sexual relationship are likely to resume satisfying sexual activity after breast cancer treatment. For some couples, the crisis of a life-threatening disease uncovers neglected problems and dissatisfactions in their relationship. Whatever the nature of their relationship, partners are likely to suffer stress and anxiety. In one study, 38% of partners questioned admitted to having sexual problems themselves, yet none had previously reported this or sought advice.

Although very many couples experience sexual problems after treatment of breast cancer, few seek help. Likewise, doctors often fail to initiate discussion of possible sexual difficulties. Women may not raise these issues because they think it is only normal to experience difficulties or because they are embarrassed to discuss them.

Reconstructive breast surgery may lessen some of the problems, particularly of self-image, but studies show that sexual problems can still persist (Weijmar Schultz et al. 1995).

Helping couples involves heightened awareness of the possibility of problems and signalling openness to discuss areas of concern. This can start during the preoperative period when possible problems and fears about sexual relations can be openly discussed with the couple. After treatment, sexual problems can develop and begin to become fixed by the third or fourth month (Anderson 1985). Counselling need not be specialist, but involves a supportive approach, encouraging couples to find joint problem-solving approaches. During the initial recovery, couples may be helped by emphasizing intimacy and a gradual return to sexual life without immediately returning to intercourse. Different positions can help to take the emphasis off the breast area, and women may prefer to make love wearing a bra and prosthesis. It may be necessary to confront myths about 'catching' cancer, being contaminated by radiation, or making cancer worse by having intercourse.

If problems persist, the couple may benefit from referral for specialist psychosexual counselling, formalizing stepwise approaches to sexual problems and perhaps exploring longer-term issues which have come to the fore after breast cancer treatment.

Case histories

Case 1

Jane a 41-year-old housewife, attends the clinic in a distraught state having just discovered that she is pregnant. She had a lumpectomy for breast cancer 5 years previously and has just discontinued her tamoxifen. She has been virtually amenorrhoeic for the last 5 years.

'I don't know what made me do a pregnancy test,' she says, 'I know I should never get pregnant again because it could make my cancer come back.'

An ultrasound scan confirms pregnancy and establishes that conception must have occurred more than a month after stopping her tamoxifen. Jane needs considerable reassurance to convince her that she is at no greater risk or recurrence of her breast cancer as a result of her pregnancy. She eventually decides to continue with the pregnancy and to request sterilization after the birth.

Case 2

Rebecca makes an urgent appointment for insertion of an intrauterine contraceptive device (IUCD). She is 18 and nulligravid and has taken COC for the last 8 months.

'My aunt has got ovarian cancer and my mum tells me both her sisters have breast cancer,' she explains, 'so I don't want to take hormones any more.'

A more detailed history reveals that the malignacies are on different sides of the family and that the affected women are more than 60 years old.

Rebecca is told that her pill will not increase her chances of breast cancer more than it does for anyone else and that it will actually reduce her chances of ovarian cancer. However, she is told that all women on the pill have a 24% increased chance of developing breast

cancer and this seems to be a very high figure to her. Despite all reassurance, she refuses any hormonal contraceptive method.

An attempt to fit an IUCD is unsuccessful because of her nulliparity. She leaves the clinic with a supply of condoms and spermicidal jelly. She promises to use these carefully and to return in the near future for a further discussion.

References

Anderson BL (1985) Sexual functioning morbidity among cancer survivors. *Cancer* 55: 1835–42.

Braendle W (1998) Hormone replacement therapy in women with breast cancer. *Anticanc Res* 18: 2253–6.

Calle EE, Martin LM, Thun MJ, Miracle HL, Heath CW (1993) Family history, age and risk of fatal breast cancer. *Am J Epidemiol* 138: 675–80.

Cauley JA, Lucas FL, Kuller LH, Vogt MT, Browner WS (1996) Bone mineral density and risk of breast cancer in older women. *JAMA* 276: 1404–8.

Colditz GA, Egan KM, Stampfer MJ (1993) Hormone replacement therapy and risk of breast cancer: results from epidemiologic studies. *Am J Obstet Gynecol* 168: 1473–80.

Colditz GA, Hankinson SE, Hunter DJ et al. (1995) The use of progestins and estrogens and the risk of breast cancer in postmenopausal women. *New Engl J Med* 332: 1589–93.

Collaborative Group on Hormonal Factors in Breast Cancer (1996) Breast cancer and hormonal contraceptives: collaborative reanalysis of individual data on 53,297 women with breast cancer and 100,239 women without breast cancer from 54 epidemiological studies. *Lancet* **347**: 1713–27.

Couch FJ, Hartmann LC (1998) BRCA1 testing—advances and retreats (editorial). *JAMA* **279**: 955–7.

DiSaia PJ, Grosen EA, Odicino F et al. (1995) Replacement therapy for breast cancer survivors. *Cancer* **76**: 2075–8.

Dixon JM, ed. (1995) *ABC of Breast Disease.* London: BMJ Publishing Group.

Dupont WD, Page DL (1991) Menopausal estrogen replacement therapy and breast cancer. *Arch Intern Med* **151**: 67–72.

Harding C, Knox WF, Faragher EB, Baildam A, Bundred NJ (1996) Hormone replacement therapy and tumour grade in breast cancer: prospective study in screening unit. *Br Med J* **312**: 1646–7.

Kroman N, Jensen MB, Melbye M, Wohlfahrt J, Mouridsen HT (1997) Should women be advised against pregnancy after breast cancer treatment? *Lancet* **350**: 319–22.

Murray PP, Stadel BV, Schlesselman JJ (1989) Oral contraceptive use in women with a family history of breast cancer. *Obstet Gynecol* **73**: 977–83.

Myers SE, Schilsky RJ (1992) Prospects for fertility after cancer chemotherapy. *Semin Oncol* **19**: 597–604.

Narod SA, Risch H, Moslehi R, Dorum A, Neuhausen S (1998) Oral contraceptives and the risk of hereditary ovarian cancer. *New Engl J Med* **339**: 424–8.

Oehninger S (1998) Will ovarian autotransplantation have a role in reproductive and gynecological medicine? *Fertil Steril* **70**: 20–21.

Royal College of Obstetricians and Gynaecologists (1997) *Pregnancy after Breast Cancer.* RCOG Guideline. London: RCOG.

Scottish Intercollegiate Guidelines Network (1998) *Breast Cancer in Women,* pp 4–5, 26. Edinburgh: SIGN Secretariat.

Spiegel D, Bloom JR, Kraemer HC, Gottheil E (1989) Effect of psychological treatment on survival of patients with metastatic breast cancer. *Lancet* **ii**: 888–91.

Surbone A, Petrek JA (1997) Childbearing issues in breast carcinoma survivors. *Cancer* **79**: 1271–8.

Thomas DB (1984) Do hormones cause breast cancer? *Cancer* **53**: 595–604.

Thomas DB (1991) Oral contraceptives and breast cancer: review of the epidemiologic literature. *Contraception* **43**: 597–642.

Ursin G, Henderson BE, Haile RW et al. (1997) Does oral contraceptive use increase the risk of breast cancer in women with BRCA1/BRCA2 mutations more than in other women? *Cancer Res* **57**: 3678–81.

Weijmar Schultz WC, Van De Wiel HBM, Hahn DEE, Wouda J (1995) Sexual adjustment of women after gynaecological and breast cancer. *Sex Marit Ther* **10**: 293–306.

WHO (1996) *Improving Access to Quality Care in Family Planning. Medical Eligibility Criteria for Contraceptive Use.* Geneva: World Health Organization.

Women with other malignant disease

Babatunde A Gbolade

2

In 1992 there was a total of 157 686 registrations of cases of cancer in females in England & Wales (Office for National Statistics 1998) with the 10 most common cancers accounting for 102 337 (*Table 1*). A diagnosis of cancer engenders fears of morbidity and mortality. Many patients have concerns about a family history of cancer because it is recognised that such a history confers one of the greatest risks of all known factors for developing cancer in an individual. However, such cancers, which are those associated with the inheritance of a mutant genetic allele and are known as hereditary cancers, constitute less than 5% of all cancer. Even in those rare families where there is an inherited predisposition to cancer, unaffected individuals have a greater than 50% chance that they will not develop an inherited cancer. Moreover, tumour clusters in families are not likely to have a significant inherited component if different organ sites are involved, if the tumours have occurred at a later date or typical age of onset, or if they have a strong environmental component, e.g. exposure to ultraviolet light. It is patients with multiple family members with tumours at the same site, early age of onset, history of multiple primary tumours and recognised associations, e.g. breast/ovary or

Table 1
The ten most common malignancies in women in England & Wales.

Malignancy	Cases registered in 1992*
Breast	31 843
Skin	20 159 (2501)**
Colorectal neoplasms	14 734
Trachea, bronchus and lung	12 327
Ovary and other uterine adnexa	5 388
Body of uterus	3 912
Stomach	3 885
Bladder	3 476
Cervix uteri	3 400
Pancreas	3 213

*Office for National Statistics 1998.
**Melanoma in parentheses.

colon/endometrial/ovarian/stomach, who may be at increased risk. Such patients need to be referred for genetic screening based on local referral criteria.

Women in the reproductive age group (15–49 years) form a significant proportion of those undergoing treatment for cancer (*Figure 1*). For such women, the spectre of reproductive cancer, including breast cancer, invariably combines their fears of morbidity and mortality with conflicts involving perceptions of their identity and sexuality. The improving long-term prospects for young cancer patients have drawn attention to the problems of fertility and contraceptive use among them. There is often the erroneous perception amongst healthcare professionals that the need for effective methods of contraception is of low priority or even non-existent in women trying to come to terms with the diagnosis of cancer. While this may be true to some extent initially, as the situation improves with treatment, many may wish to resume sexual activity.

Treatment for genital tract cancers often, but not always, involves extirpation of the reproductive organs such that there will be no further pregnancies. Where treatment has not resulted in removal of the reproductive organs and there is the desire to maintain fertility with a view to a future pregnancy, appropriate methods of contraception need to be provided.

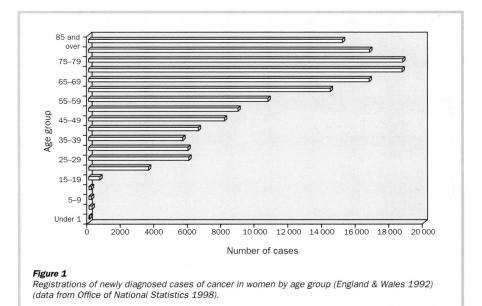

Figure 1
Registrations of newly diagnosed cases of cancer in women by age group (England & Wales 1992)
(data from Office of National Statistics 1998).

The timing of pregnancy is an important issue in women with a malignancy

Timing is particularly important if irradiation or chemotherapy are treatment options. Family planning becomes crucial in the overall management of these patients. Lomax (Family Planning Nurse Instructors' Project, unpublished data) surveyed 35 United Kingdom oncology centres. She found that although 34 respondents felt there was a need for contraceptive advice in women undergoing chemotherapy, no method was prescribed in 14 centres. Although doctors and nurses in 34 centres provided contraceptive advice, only in one centre had the adviser undergone formal training in family planning. Thirteen respondents were aware of patients who had undergone termination of an unplanned pregnancy while undergoing chemotherapy.

The importance of contraception during cytotoxic chemotherapy cannot be overemphasized

Many cytotoxic drugs used are teratogenic and mutagenic. Fetal conception during toxic chemotherapy may result in abortion of the embryo, or in gross congenital abnormalities of the fetus. Hence termination of the pregnancy is usually recommended if chemotherapy has to be given during early pregnancy. Many chemotherapeutic agents also interfere with ovarian or other reproductive functions, the effects depending on the cumulative dose, duration of treatment and patient's age especially in relation to puberty (prepubertal patients being less susceptible). Chemotherapy may result in infertility especially if high-dose alkylating agents are used in pubertal and older women. Preservation of ova or ovaries is not widely available.

If fertility is a possibility, the patient should be advised to avoid conception for at least a year after completion of chemotherapy

While long-term survivors of cancer therapy have not shown evidence of increased rates of stillbirths, fetal abnormalities or spontaneous abortion (Goldman and Johnson 1993), very little has been published in the literature on the use of contraceptive methods in patients with cancer. The literature is also scarce on the effect of any contraceptive device, including hormonal contraceptives, on malignancies.

When giving contraceptive advice to patients with cancer, either cured, in remission or currently undergoing treatment, due consideration needs to be given to the reliability and compliance of the individual. A major problem is determining the duration of medical contraindication of pregnancy after cancer treatment, the decision depending largely on the risk of relapse or metastasis. Also, the risks of an unplanned pregnancy have to be balanced against the risks associated with use of the contraceptive method either on its own or in relation to the type of cancer and the treatment. The hormone dependency or receptor status of the different cancers, possible drug interactions and side effects of treatment modalities also influence the choice of contraceptive method. In most cases, the use of barrier methods or male sterilization should be suitable. However, these methods may not be acceptable to some individuals.

Genital malignancies

Ovarian cancer

Ovarian cancer affects around 5000 women in the United Kingdom resulting in about 4000 deaths annually. While the disease is seen more in women over the age of 40 years, it is not unknown to occur in younger women. Women with advanced ovarian cancer would usually undergo extensive surgery involving removal of the uterus and ovaries in which case there would be no need for contraception. In early stage disease, chemotherapy and radiotherapy may result in ovarian failure (Shalet 1980) although normal pregnancies following chemotherapy have been reported (Schneider et al. 1988, Lee et al. 1989). Unilateral oophorectomy may be carried out in a young woman with stage 1A grade 1 ovarian cancer where conservation of fertility is desired. Although combined oral contraceptives have a protective effect on the incidence of epithelial ovarian cancers, we have found no data on the effect of oral contraceptive pills on recurrence rates in women who have had conservative treatment. The presence of oestrogen and progestogen receptors in ovarian cancer tissue is frequently related to the grade of the tumour (Kaupilla et al. 1983). Since combined oral contraceptive pills and depot medroxyprogesterone acetate work mainly by ovulation suppression, it is probably safe to use them in this group of women. In situations where the hormone dependency status of the tumour remains in doubt, the intrauterine device (IUD), barrier methods and natural methods of contraception would appear to be the best and most suitable although efficacy is less in the last two. The levonorgestrel-releasing IUD may be used if the tumour is not hormone dependent.

Cervical cancer

Reliable data on the use or non-use of hormonal contraceptives by women with cervical cancer are sorely lacking. Few women who have had treatment for malignancies of the cervix retain their fertility and there does not appear to be any published studies concerning the risk of recurrence of cervical cancer and current use of hormonal contraceptives. More women treated successfully for premalignant disease of the cervix generally retain their reproductive potential and can use any type of contraception including hormonal methods (IPPF 1999). A further area of concern is the advisability of the use of hormonal contraceptives in women with current cervical dysplasia. From the available published studies, there is no strong evidence to warrant withholding use in these women. Inadvertent pregnancy while undergoing investigations will entail more difficulties for the woman and her doctor. However, further studies are needed.

All forms of hormonal contraceptives can be given to women with a family history of cervical cancer

Choriocarcinoma

Choriocarcinoma, a malignant tumour, may follow a hydatidiform mole, an abortion or a normal pregnancy. In the UK, it occurs in 1 in 30 000 pregnancies. While on the whole, tumour size and the interval between the antecedent pregnancy and the commencement of chemotherapy determine survival and cure rates, delay in diagnosis may lead to treatment failure (Vartiainen et al. 1998). Pregnancy after successful treatment of choriocarcinoma can and does occur (O'Neill et al. 1976); therefore, an unplanned pregnancy should be prevented by use of an effective method of contraception. It is recommended that pregnancy be avoided for 12 months after completing chemotherapy so that elimination of the disease can be confirmed and risk of teratogenicity from the chemotherapy minimised (Newlands 1995). The use of progestogen-only implants, copper IUDs and levonorgestrel-containing IUDs is contraindicated in women receiving treatment for choriocarcinoma or during follow-up

because they often cause heavy or irregular bleeding. This may give rise to confusion (Vartiainen et al. 1998), as vaginal bleeding is an important symptom of recurrence. The combined oral contraceptive pill provides efficient contraception and suppresses pituitary luteinizing hormone (LH) which may cross-react with human chorionic gonadotrophin (hCG) in less specific assays. However, Stone and colleagues (1976) reported that using combined oral contraceptives delayed the fall in hCG in women who had a hydatidiform mole but did not need chemotherapy. According to him, oral contraceptives also increased the need for chemotherapy for trophoblastic tumour after evacuation of a hydatidiform mole in women taking the pill before normal hCG values were obtained. The relevance of this finding to choriocarcinoma is not known, nor is it clear whether oral contraceptives increase the risk of trophoblastic disease itself or of postmolar malignant transformation. However, other studies (Berkowitz et al. 1981, Curry et al. 1989, Deicas et al. 1991) have not confirmed this finding.

Hormonal methods should be avoided until the beta-hCG levels are back to normal

The advice from Newlands (1994) is that oral contraceptives should be avoided until beta-HCG levels have been back to normal for at least six months, unless the patient is unlikely to comply with interim use of barrier or natural methods.

Non-genital malignancies

Breast cancer

The risk of developing new breast cancer is greatest in women with a previous history and about 7% of women who have undergone mastectomy will have one or more pregnancies subsequently. As the risk of recurrence is greatest during the first three years it is recommended that pregnancy should be delayed beyond that time (Horstein et al. 1982). Tamoxifen, as adjuvant therapy, is beneficial in premenopausal women with a relative 12% reduction in the annual risk of recurrence and 6% reduction in mortality (Early Breast Cancer Trialists Collaboration Group 1992). However, its partial oestrogenic agonist effect often induces endometrial hyperplasia and can cause uterine cancer (Neven et al. 1994). Theoretically, this effect can be countered and contraception obtained by the use of the levonorgestrel-releasing IUD. There are ongoing studies to determine the effectiveness of this device in the prevention and treatment of endometrial hyperplasia in this situation. Because of the possibility of oestrogen dependency in women with a history of breast cancer, hormonal therapy would not be advisable in these women or in women with a known oestrogen-dependent tumour. In effect, combined oral contraceptive pills and combined injectable contraceptives are contraindicated but the copper IUD and barrier methods may be used.

Hodgkin's disease and non-Hodgkin's lymphoma

Irradiation is the primary modality of treatment for the majority of localized stages of Hodgkin's disease, i.e. stages 1, 2 and some 3A. Chemotherapy may be used in addition to irradiation when apparently localized disease is associated with adverse prognostic factors. Temporary menstrual dysfunction is common and may lead to unplanned pregnancy if adequate contraception is not used, although pregnancy does not appear to accelerate Hodgkin's disease or to affect survival adversely (Thomas and Peckham 1976). Oral contraceptives have been shown to protect ovarian function in women receiving chemotherapy for Hodgkin's disease (Chapman and Sutcliffe 1981). Long-term remission may follow treatment of disseminated Hodgkin's disease with combination chemotherapy (Rosenberg and Kaplan 1975). Because the majority of relapses will occur within two years, patients with active disease are usually advised to avoid pregnancy and wait until the disease has been quiescent for this period. During the waiting period, virtually all methods of contraception including the combined oral contraceptive pill may be used. These same considerations apply to non-Hodgkin's lymphoma.

Malignant melanoma

Malignant melanoma is often diagnosed in women of childbearing age and may run an unpredictable course. Previously, pregnancy was regarded as an unfavourable prognostic factor in women with this disease and termination of pregnancy used to be recommended. The situation appears to have changed (Slingluff and Reintgen 1993) but because the first two to three years after diagnosis is the period with the highest probability of relapse, prudence dictates that pregnancy should be avoided during this period. The use of oral contraceptives does not appear to be contraindicated in melanoma patients (Osterlind and colleagues 1988), but the side effects of chemotherapy and radiotherapy which often result in severe vomiting and nausea, may preclude their use in certain groups of patients. Other suitable methods of contraception including barrier methods, IUDs and injectables may be used.

The leukaemias

Women with a history of current or previous treatment for leukaemia will have different problems depending on the type. Subsequent fertility depends on the type of chemotherapy regimen used as some are more likely to cause ovarian failure than others. Radiation also may produce ovarian failure unless the ovaries are shielded. Severe problems with menorrhagia may occur because of thrombocytopenia complicating the malignancy or chemotherapy. Those who remain fertile may use barrier methods or combined oral contraceptive pills.

Thrombocytopenia precludes the use of the progestogen-only pill, implants and copper IUDs

This is because of the potential side effects of irregular bleeding or menorrhagia (Howard and Tuck 1995). However, the levonorgestrel-releasing IUD or depot medroxyprogesterone acetate may improve menorrhagia after initial irregular bleeding.

Liver cancer

Combined oral contraceptives are contraindicated in patients with liver cancer and although progestogen-only pills do not noticeably affect liver metabolism, a non-hormonal method should be the first choice.

Meningioma

Meningiomas are twice as frequent in females compared with males. They have been shown to have steroid hormone receptors, especially progesterone receptors (Grunberg et al. 1991) and to be affected by pregnancy. In women with such tumours, prudence dictates that steroid hormonal contraceptives should be avoided.

Conclusion

Because most cancers in women occur at a stage well beyond the reproductive age, there is lack of information about appropriate contraceptive methods for women in the reproductive age group with a diagnosis of cancer. Many patients may suffer permanent reproductive failure because the effects of cytotoxic agents or radiotherapy on female germ cells are variable and idiosyncratic. In most cases where the capacity for reproduction is preserved, the use of barrier methods (although less effective) or male sterilization would address the issue of contraception satisfactorily. For some individuals, these methods may not be acceptable. Women with non-oestrogen-dependent tumours may use hormonal contraceptives. Termination of a pregnancy may be advisable if the woman has undergone chemotherapy or irradiation in the first trimester. In view of the limited literature dealing with this area, we have presented what we think is a reasonable approach to managing these women. However, this may change in the light of new evidence in future.

Case histories

Case 1

Judy was a 22-year-old normally menstruating nullipara, who had complained of intermittent long-standing pelvic pain. She was found at laparotomy to have a left ovarian tumour with ascites. There were no palpable lymph nodes, omental or liver metastasis. Left salpingo-oophorectomy and biopsy of the enlarged right ovary was performed.
Histopathology report showed endometroid adenocarcinoma of the left ovary but the right ovary was normal. There were malignant cells in the ascitic fluid. She subsequently was treated with combination chemotherapy with Cisplatinum and Adriamycin followed by maintenance chemotherapy with Treosulfan which was discontinued 13 months later as examination did not reveal any evidence of a pelvic mass. Judy became pregnant with twins a month later. The pregnancy progressed uneventfully and she was delivered by elective caesarean section at 38 weeks. She subsequently used combined oral contraceptive pills. She had regular follow ups until she was discovered to have a right-sided adnexal mass suggestive of ovarian cancer and uterine enlargement five years later. Total abdominal

hysterectomy and right salpingo-oopherectomy along with peritoneal washes and lymph-node biopsies were performed. None of these showed any evidence of malignancy at histology and cytology. At the present time Judy remains well and free of disease.

Case 2

Toni, a 26-year-old woman, about to get married, was diagnosed with Hodgkin's lymphoma. In the course of discussions about her management, she expressed a very strong desire to have children. She was told that following chemotherapy for Hodgkin's disease, young women tend to become prematurely menopausal. Pretreatment biopsy of her ovaries showed the presence of an average of 12 primordial and primary follicles per 5 × 5 mm biopsy section. In order to avoid pregnancy during the full course of MVPP (mechlorethamine, vinblastine, procarbazine, prednisone) therapy, she used the combined oral contraceptive pill. Her post-treatment ovarian biopsy tissue showed more than 25 follicles per histologic section. She discontinued use of the combined oral contraceptive pill 28 months following chemotherapy and resumed normal menstruation a month

later. Toni became pregnant seven months after discontinuing use of the combined oral contraceptive pill and had an uneventful pregnancy and delivery.

References

Berkowitz RS, Goldstein DP, Marean ER, Bernstein M (1981) Oral contraceptives and postmolar trophoblastic disease. *Obstet Gynecol* **58**: 474–7.

Chapman RM, Sutcliffe SB (1981) Protection of ovarian function by oral contraceptives in women receiving chemotherapy for Hodgkin's disease. *Blood* **58**: 849–51.

Curry SL, Schlaert JB, Kohorn EI et al. (1989) Hormonal contraception and trophoblastic sequelae after hydatidiform mole (A Gynaecologic Oncology Group Study). *Am J Obstet Gynecol* **160**: 805–11.

Deicas RE, Miller DS, Rademaker AW, Lurain JR (1991) The role of contraception in the development of post-molar gestational trophoblastic disease. *Obstet Gynecol* **78**: 221–6.

Early Breast Cancer Trialists Collaboration Group (1992) Systemic treatment of early breast cancer by hormonal, cytotoxic or immune therapy. *Lancet* **339**: 1–25.

Goldman S, Johnson FL (1993) Effects of chemotherapy and irradiation of the gonads. *Adolescent Endocrinol* **22**: 617–29.

Grunberg SM, Weiss MH, Spitz IM et al. (1991) Treatment of unresectable meningiomas with the antiprogesterone agent mifepristone. *J Neurosurg* **74**: 861–6.

Hornstein E, Skornick Y, Rozin R (1982) The management of breast carcinoma in pregnancy and lactation. *J Surg Oncol* **21**: 179–82.

Howard RJ, Tuck SM (1995) Haematological disorders and reproductive health. *Br J Fam Plann* **19**: 147–50.

International Planned Parenthood Federation (1999) IMAP statement on contraception for women with medical disorders. *IPPF Med Bull* **33**(5): 2.

Kaupilla A, Vierriko P, Kivinen S et al. (1983) Clinical significance of estrogen and progestin in ovarian cancer. *Obstet Gynecol* **61**: 320–6.

Lee RB, Kelly J, Elg SA, Benson WL (1989) Pregnancy following conservative surgery and adjunctive chemotherapy for stage III immature tertoma of the ovary. *Obstet Gynecol* **73**: 853–5.

Neven P, De Muylder X, Van Belle Y et al. (1994) Tamoxifen and the uterus. *Br Med J* **309**: 1313–4.

Newlands ES (1994) Trophoblastic disease and hormones. *Br J Fam Plann* **19**: 276–7.

Newlands ES (1995) Clinical management of trophoblastic disease in the United Kingdom. *Current Obstet Gynaecol* **5**: 19–24.

Office of National Statistics (1998) *Cancer Statistics Registrations (1992), England & Wales.* Series MB1, no. 25. London: The Stationery Office.

O'Neill E, Pelegrina I, Hammond CB et al. (1976) Normal pregnancy and delivery after cerebral metastasis of choriocarcinoma. *Cancer* **38**: 984–6.

Osterlind A, Tucker MA, Stone BJ, Jansen OM (1988) The Danish case-control study of cutaneous malignant melanoma III. Hormonal and reproductive factors in women. *Int J Cancer* **42**: 821–4.

Rosenberg SA, Kaplan HS (1975) The management of stages I, II and III Hodgkin's disease with combined radiotherapy and chemotherapy. *Cancer* **35**: 55–63.

Schneider J, Erasun F, Hervas JL et al. (1988) Normal pregnancy and delivery two years after adjuvant chemotherapy for grade III immature ovarian teratoma. *Gynecol Oncol* **29**: 245–9.

Shalet S (1980) Effects of cancer chemotherapy on gonadal function of patients with cancer. *Cancer Treat Rev* **7**: 141–52.

Slinguff CL Jr, Reintgen D (1993) Malignant melanoma and the prognostic implications of pregnancy, oral contraceptives and exogenous hormones. *Semin Surg Oncol* **9**: 228–31.

Stone M, Dent J, Kardana A, Bagshawe KD (1976) Relationship of oral contraception to development of trophoblastic tumour after evacuation of a hydatidiform mole. *Br J Obst Gynaecol* **83**: 913–16.

Thomas PRM, Peckham MJ (1976) The investigation and management of Hodgkin's disease in the pregnant patient. *Cancer* **38**: 1443–56.

Vartiainen J, Alfthan H, Lehtovirta P, Stenman UH (1998) Identification of choriocarcinoma by the hCG beta-to-hCG proportion in patients with delayed diagnosis caused by contraceptive use. *Contraception* **57**: 257–60.

Women at risk of venous thromboembolism

Anne Szarewski

3

Venous thromboembolism (VTE) essentially encompasses deep vein thrombosis (DVT) of the legs, pulmonary embolism (PE) and cerebral sinus thrombosis (CST). It is rare in the general population, but the incidence rises with age, from 1 per 100 000 people per year in childhood to nearly 1% per year in old age (Rosendaal 1999). Specifically in women aged 15 to 49 years it has been estimated that the overall incidence of DVT is 21 per 100 000 women per year (Vandenbroucke 1996). In pregnancy, the risk of antenatal DVT is about 61 per 100 000 in women under the age of 35 and 121 per 100 000 in women over that age. The rate of postpartum DVT is about 30 per 100 000 in women under the age of 35 and 72 per 100 000 in older women (Greer 1999). Of those who suffer a DVT, 1–2% will die, usually owing to a pulmonary embolism.

Risk factors for venous thromboembolism

Venous thrombosis results from a combination of inherited and acquired risk factors (*Figure 1*).

Figure 1
Risk factors for venous thromboembolism

Inherited

Antithrombin deficiency
Protein C deficiency
Protein S deficiency
Activated protein C resistance, factor V Leiden mutation
Factor XII deficiency

Acquired

Immobility
Surgery, trauma
Obesity
Pregnancy/pueperium
Long distance travel
Use of combined oral contraceptives/hormone replacement therapy
Antiphospholipid antibody, lupus anticoagulant
Malignancy
?Smoking (see text)
?Varicose veins (see text)

The role of inherited thrombophilias has been increasingly recognized during the last decade.

It is now possible to identify a genetic contribution in approximately half the patients who present with a first DVT, and new genetic coagulation disorders are being discovered all the time.

There is probably a genetic contribution to most cases of DVT

The coagulation system is constantly balancing the effects of procoagulants and anticoagulants. The major anticoagulant factors are:

1. antithrombin, which neutralizes thrombin and other procoagulant enzymes

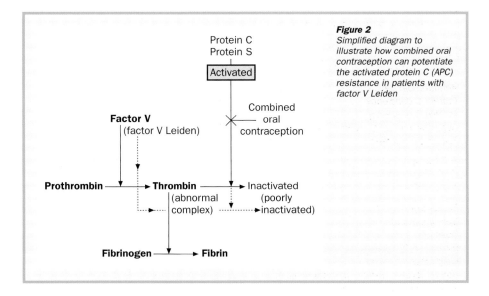

Figure 2
Simplified diagram to illustrate how combined oral contraception can potentiate the activated protein C (APC) resistance in patients with factor V Leiden

2. protein C, which inactivates cofactors V and VIII

3. protein S, the cofactor for protein C

4. thrombomodulin, which enables thrombin to activate protein C

The classic thrombophilias are the ones arising from a deficiency of antithrombin, protein C or protein S. These cause an estimated 20-fold increase in the risk of thrombosis, but in absolute terms are rare, accounting for no more than 8% of patients investigated after a first thrombosis (Laffan et al. 1998).

However, the major breakthrough in this area was the discovery of factor V Leiden mutation in 1994 (Bertina et al. 1994). The mutated form of factor V is resistant to inactivation by protein C; since protein C is an anticoagulant (see above), the result is an increased tendency to thrombosis. This scenario is known as activated protein C (APC) resistance (*Figure 2*).

Factor V Leiden is found in approximately 5% of Caucasians, though higher rates (15%) have been found in some populations, for example in Sweden and Greece (Vandenbroucke et al. 1996). However, the

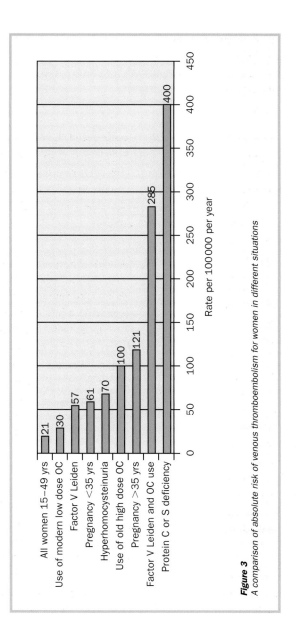

Figure 3

A comparison of absolute risk of venous thromboembolism for women in different situations

prevalence appears to be extremely low in African and Oriental women. The mutation is found in 20% of patients with VTE; among carriers, the risk of thrombosis is 57 per 100 000 women per year.

Since the discovery of factor V Leiden, several other genetic mutations have come to light, including another factor V variant (factor V Cambridge) and a prothrombin gene mutation (prothrombin 20210A), which was found in 18% of patients who had suffered a VTE (Provan et al. 1999) but in only 1–2% of normal control subjects.

More complex genetic changes can result in abnormally high levels of clotting factors. This has been shown to be the explanation for the relatively increased risk of thrombosis in people with blood groups other than O, who have higher levels of clotting factor VIII. Factor VIII concentrations that exceed 1500 IU/l (150% of normal) have been found in 11% of the general population and 25% of patients with thrombosis. Such high concentrations were associated with a six-fold increase in the risk of thrombosis. Another example is that of hyperhomocysteinuria, whose sufferers have an increased risk (three- to four-fold) of thrombosis (Rosendaal 1999) (*Figure 3*).

However, it is important to remember that one inherited defect of coagulation is unlikely to result in a VTE on its own.

A single inherited defect is unlikely to be the sole cause of VTE

It is frequently found that individuals with thrombophilia have several genetic coagulation defects at the same time. And even then, they are likely to require another, acquired risk factor, before thrombosis occurs.

Acquired risk factors, such as pregnancy, immobilization and use of combined oral contraceptives are common. It is also often forgotten that increasing age is in itself a risk factor for thrombosis, and this is unavoidable. A feature which is common to thrombophilic families is that the mean age at first thrombosis is much younger than for consecutive patients with thrombosis, irrespective of the underlying defect and even when no defect has been identified (*Figure 4*).

A synergistic effect has been shown for factor V Leiden and combined oral contraceptive (COC) use. Women who use COCs but are not carriers of factor V Leiden have a risk of VTE of around 30 per 100 000 per year. The risk for carriers of the defect who do not use COCs is 57 per 100 000 per year. However, for women who are carriers and use COCs,

Figure 4
Age at first thrombosis by origin of patient

Risk factor	Age (years) at first thrombosis	
	Patients from thrombophilic families (n = 78)	Consecutive unselected patients (n = 105)
Protein C deficiency	31	47
Factor V Leiden	29	43
No defect found	34	46

*Reproduced with permission from Rosendaal FR, Lancet 1999; **353**: 1167–73.*

the risk jumps to 285 per 100 000 per year (Vandenbroucke et al. 1996).

Similarly, COC use and the presence of coagulation defects leads to much higher risks of cerebral sinus thrombosis (30 to 150 times) than found in women who use COCs but do not have a thrombophilia (de Bruijn et al. 1998, Martinelli et al. 1998).

The combined oral contraceptive pill and venous thrombosis

The first definite link between the combined pill and venous thrombosis was made by the Royal College of General Practitioners' Study (RCGP 1967) and that of Vessey and Doll in 1968. At the time, the risk of VTE with these high dose pills was estimated at 100 per 100 000 women per year (Vessey 1989). The risk of VTE was found to be dependent on the dose of oestrogen in the pill (Inman 1970), and this was subsequently reduced. Studies which later looked at the risk of VTE with second generation (30–35 µg ethinyloestradiol) pills found risks of 39 and 42 per 100 000 women per year (Vessey 1986; Stadel 1981; Gerstman et al. 1991).

In October 1995, the United Kingdom Committee on Safety of Medicines (CSM) released a 'Dear Doctor' letter, warning doctors about an increased risk of venous thromboembolism in women taking third generation COC pills. These pills, containing the progestogens desogestrel and gestodene, had been on the market since the mid-1980s and were extremely popular. It has been estimated that in 1995 approximately 1.5 million women in the UK were taking this type of pill.

The papers on which the CSM based their advice were not published until later that year and the next year (Jick 1995; WHO 1995; Spitzer et al. 1996), resulting in considerable confusion. This was the first time that it had been suggested that a difference in progestogen type could so greatly influence venous thromboembolic risk, which had previously always been attributed to oestrogen.

The new studies showed a risk of VTE for users of third generation pills of 30 per 100 000 women per year, which is in fact a slightly lower figure than that shown in previous studies for second generation pills. However, in these studies the risk for second generation pills had dropped to 15 per 100 000 women per year. The CSM therefore stated that there was a doubling of risk for users of third generation pills and advised doctors that desogestrel and gestodene-containing pills should no longer routinely be used as first choice contraceptives.

Many doctors believe that regulatory action was unnecessary in 1995, and that the way in which it was carried out, prior to publication of the studies, was irresponsible (Spitzer 1997, Edwards 1997, Benagiano 1998, Cohen 1998, Spitzer 1998, Mills 1999, Szarewski and Mansour 1999). None of the studies was beyond criticism and there has been much debate about the role of prescribing bias and confounding factors as possible explanations for the apparent increase in risk for third generation pills.

The most obvious example of prescriber bias can be seen with the Mercilon–Marvelon paradox. Mercilon and Marvelon both contain the same amount (150 µg) of desogestrel, but in Marvelon this is combined with 30 µg ethinyloestradiol, while in Mercilon the oestrogen dose is lower, at 20 µg. It would therefore seem self-evident that the risk of VTE should be lower in users of Mercilon, and yet in all the recent studies, risks for VTE have been higher in users of Mercilon. Clearly, doctors were prescribing the lower dose product to women considered at higher risk (e.g. because of family history or obesity). This whole issue has been well summarized by Spitzer (1997).

An appeal was mounted against the CSM's decision, finally being heard by the Medicines Commission (an independent body) in November 1998. Studies published since 1995 were presented to the Commission (Farmer 1997, Suissa 1997, Lidegaard 1998), as was a large UK GP database study which is still awaiting publication (Farmer et al. 2000). Newer studies, which have been better able to take prescriber bias and confounding into account, tend to show no significant difference between second and third generation pills.

In April 1999, as a result of the Medicines Commission appeal, the Department of Health announced an end to the 1995 restrictions on prescribing third generation pills (Department of Health 1999, Medicines Control Agency 1999), stating that 'The absolute risk of VTE in women taking third generation COCs is very small and is much less than the risk in pregnancy' and 'provided women are fully informed of these very small risks and do not have medical contraindications, it should be a matter of clinical judgement and personal choice which type of oral contraceptive should be prescribed.' The effect of this is that third generation pills can be prescribed as first line again. A similar appeal has been successful in Germany.

The data sheets of gestodene and desogestrel-containing pills in the UK will, however, carry a new wording, stating that these types of pill carry a risk of VTE of 'about 25 per 100 000 women per year', while for second generation pills, the risk is 'about 15 per 100 000 women per year.'

Third generation pills have benefits in terms of quality of life (CPMP 1996), but this aspect is, unfortunately, difficult to quantify. Third generation progestogens, while still giving good cycle control, are less androgenic than second generation products and therefore tend to be better for women who have problems with acne, hirsutism, and weight gain (Guillebaud 1995, Clinical and Scientific Committee 1995, Le Blanc and Laws 1999). These are termed 'minor' side effects, but have been shown to greatly influence compliance (International Working Group on Enhancing Patient Compliance and Oral Contraceptive Efficacy 1993). It is noteworthy that a norgestimate-containing pill (which was not evaluated in the three studies of VTE risk) has recently been licensed by the United States Food and Drug Administration for the treatment of acne, having been proved effective in a randomized placebo-controlled trial (Redmond 1997). Further scientific studies of other third generation pills are needed to clarify the anecdotal reports of their beneficial effects.

There is some evidence that third generation COCs may be safer for women at risk of arterial disease, which would add another layer to the risk–benefit analysis, since some risk factors for both arterial and venous disease overlap. Of particular interest is that in the latest study by Farmer et al. (2000) smoking, which has previously been viewed as a purely arterial risk factor, was found to be a significant risk factor for VTE (OR 2.0, 95% CI 1.4–2.7). One study has shown a statistically significant reduction in risk of myocardial infarction (MI) in users of desogestrel and gestodene-containing pills, compared with second generation products (Lewis 1997). The WHO study has shown results consistent with this for stroke, but did not reach statistical significance (Poulter 1999), while a third study failed to show a difference between the two types of pill for MI (Dunn 1999).

Prescribing implications

Clearly, women who have already had a venous thrombosis should not be prescribed oestrogen-containing oral contraceptives, of any kind (Mills et al. 1998). The question has been raised as to whether all women considering the COC should be screened for thrombophilias. The answer is an unequivocal 'no'. It has been estimated that screening one million women would prevent one death per year from VTE (Mills 1998). However, there is considerable debate around the issue of women who have a family history of VTE. Although, again, relatively few lives may be saved (four women per million screened), there is a consensus that this may be worthwhile for the individual.

Women with a strong family history of VTE should be screened prior to oral contraceptive use

What constitutes a family history? The strongest case can be made for a definite (proven) history of VTE in a first degree relative under the age of 45. However, since women who are about to take the pill for the first time are likely to be young, their first degree relatives may well not yet have had their VTE, the risk of which increases with age. Also, with family size becoming smaller, they may not have siblings at all. Stretching the criteria to include more distant relatives will certainly detect more cases, but at the cost of worrying a large number of women unnecessarily. A major problem with screening is that currently, even in people who have had a VTE, a coagulation defect can only be detected in about 50% (Hampton et al. 1997). This means that a negative screen does not give complete reassurance; only a few years ago, all the women now known to be positive for factor V Leiden, with their greatly increased risk, would have been told they were 'clear'. This situation is likely to improve in the future, as more coagulation defects are recognized and the tests become simpler (and therefore cheaper to do 'en masse').

It is clear that screening for only one coagulation defect is not very useful: if screening is to be done at all, a bank of tests is required. This should include assays of fibrinogen, antithrombin III, protein C, protein S, activated protein C resistance, antiphospholipid antibodies and factor V

Leiden (Machin 1995). It seems to be a general principle in haemostatic screening that more is better. If all these tests are negative, the woman should still be advised that the thrombophilia cannot be absolutely excluded, but, on this understanding, if she wishes to take the COC, it can be prescribed. However, it should not be forgotten that the reverse scenario is also true: many women found to have a thrombophilia will not in fact go on to develop a VTE and will therefore have been worried and may have avoided the pill unnecessarily. It should also be borne in mind that the greatest risk of VTE occurs in the first year of pill use (Spitzer 1997): thus, if a woman has already been on the pill for over a year (without having developed a VTE), she is likely to be at reduced risk.

Other risk factors and the COC

Since VTE is a multifactorial problem, even women without a family history may have risk factors which make taking the combined pill inadvisable. One of the most important of these is obesity, specifically a body mass index (BMI) of over 30 kg/m².

In the study by Farmer et al. (2000), women with a BMI over 35 kg/m² were at four times the risk of VTE compared with women whose BMI was 20–25 kg/m².

It is often assumed that women with varicose veins should be cautious about taking the pill,

but this is not substantiated (Campbell 1996). However, women should be reminded to stop taking the pill about four weeks prior to major surgery or immobilization and not to resume for the same length of time afterwards (Guillebaud 1989).

Obese women have four times the risk of VTE

Should first time users and women with a family history of VTE (and negative screen) be prescribed second or third generation pills as first choice?

Since the revision of the 1995 CSM guidelines, this is now a matter for the doctor and the individual woman, based on the risks and benefits of a particular pill in her case. Women should be made aware of the risks of VTE, as presented in the new data sheets. Personally, I do not believe that second generation pills can have become safer over a ten year period: there has, after all, not been any change in their formulation. I therefore tell women that the risk of VTE with all combined pills is around 30 per 100 000 women per year (i.e. the figure which has been quoted since the studies of low dose pills in the 1980s, and the higher figure from the new studies). If this level of risk is greater than they wish to take, then I do not feel I can honestly reassure them that one type of pill is likely to be safer than another in their case, and I suggest they consider an alternative method of contraception.

What about Cilest and Dianette?

Cilest (35 µg ethinyloestradiol plus 250 µg norgestimate) and Dianette (35 µg ethinyloestradiol plus 2 mg cyproterone acetate) were not evaluated in the studies on which the CSM based their guidelines in 1995. The restrictions on prescribing have therefore never applied to these pills, and they are unaffected by the changes in the data sheets for desogestrel and gestodene-containing pills.

Other contraceptive options

If the woman cannot, or does not wish to use the combined pill, there are still many options open to her. However, it should be remembered that pregnancy also poses a very significant risk of VTE, and therefore the method chosen should preferably be very effective at preventing pregnancy.

Progestogen-only methods are all suitable for women at risk of VTE, as progestogen on its own has not been demonstrated to have any significant effects on coagulation. Nor has it been associated with VTE in epidemiological studies (Fotherby 1989a, Machin et al. 1995). Progestogen-only pills (Broome and Macauley 1996, Fotherby 1989b), injectable progestogens (Lande 1995), implants (Davies and Newton 1991, Machin et al. 1995, Egberg et al. 1998) and the intrauterine levonorgestrel-releasing system (Luukkainen 1991) are all possible choices. Of these, the progestogen-only pill (POP) is somewhat less effective in young women (Fotherby 1989a,b), with failure rates of around 4 per hundred woman years. By the age of 35, however, its efficacy is equivalent to that of the combined pill, at less than one per hundred woman-years. All the other progestogen-only methods have very low failure rates (less than one per hundred woman-years) and have the advantage that they are all long-acting, requiring little effort on the part of the user. However, all (including the POP) have the side effect of causing irregularity of menstruation.

Depomedroxyprogesterone acetate has a particular advantage in women with sickle cell disease (with its higher risk of thrombosis), as it has been shown to reduce the number of crises and improve the haematological picture (Lande 1995).

DMPA reduces the number of sickle cell crises

Although women at risk of VTE can use oestrogen-containing hormonal emergency contraception (the Yuzpe regimen, or PC4), there is now an option which should be safer, since it contains only progestogen (WHO 1998). A randomized trial showed a failure rate of only 1.1% (95% CI 0.6–2.0). As well as being more effective than Yuzpe, the levonorgestrel regimen was associated with significantly fewer side effects, particularly nausea (23% vs 51%, $p < 0.01$) and vomiting (6% vs 19%, $p < 0.01$).

The levonorgestrel regimen is now licensed for post-coital use in the UK. Levonelle-2 consists of two tablets, each of 750 µg of levonorgestrel. The first tablet should be taken within 72 hours of unprotected intercourse, and the second 12 hours later. Interestingly, research has shown that the efficacy is greater, the earlier the first tablet is taken. Alternatively the dosage can be given using POP (40 tablets of Neogest, 50 tablets of Microval or 50 tablets of Norgeston, split into two doses, 12 hours apart).

All the non-hormonal methods are theoretically suitable, although barrier methods and natural family planning may have unacceptably high failure rates. Modern copper intrauterine devices (e.g. the Copper T 380, the Gynefix) are extremely effective, with failure rates of less than one per hundred woman-years.

Conclusion

Women at risk of venous thrombosis have a wider choice of contraceptive methods than they (and their doctors) often think. History taking is important in order to elucidate familial risk as well as other potential risk factors. It should be remembered that VTE is a multifactorial disease, usually the result of an interaction between several risk factors, both genetic and acquired. In the future, screening of thrombophilia should become a better predictor of risk, as more coagulation defects are discovered and tests become simpler, cheaper and more comprehensive. In the interim, women at risk are in particular need of information to enable them to make what are often difficult decisions.

Case histories

Case 1

Diana is a 38-year-old clerk who smokes 20 cigarettes per day. Many years ago, when she first started taking the combined pill, she had a DVT. She was advised not to take the COC any more, and tried the progestogen-only pill. However, she found the strict time-keeping too difficult and decided since she wasn't taking it properly she might as well stop. She then tried an IUD, but had it removed, because of 'an infection' (she couldn't remember quite what it was). She and her boyfriend had been using condoms, but he didn't like them. Recently, he was treated for 'something' in a clinic, but she had no symptoms. She had a termination of pregnancy nine months ago.

'I never want to go through anything like that again,' she says.

A long discussion ensues regarding her contraceptive options. A long-acting progestogen-only method could be ideal. She is not sure about Depo-Provera (depot medroxyprogesterone acetate) because she feels she might want a baby in the next couple of years and is worried about the possibility of a delay in return of fertility. An implant is a possibility, with the advantage of rapid reversibility. However, she feels a little squeamish about the idea and is not too sure about the side effect of irregular bleeding (on balance, she prefers the idea of amenorrhoea with Depo-Provera).

The idea of a Mirena (intrauterine system) is discussed. Clearly, this would not be ideal because of the possible history of pelvic inflammatory disease (PID), but since the Mirena does not

appear to increase the risk of PID, it could be considered. A screen for sexually transmitted disease would be necessary, and fitting would probably be best done under antibiotic cover.

The diaphragm is also briefly discussed, but she does not like the idea and feels that the higher failure rate does not merit the extra effort involved.

After thinking it over, and discussing it with her boyfriend, she decides to have Implanon (a desogestrel-releasing implant) fitted.

This has so far been successful, especially since her periods have been reasonably regular.

Case 2

Margaret is an air hostess, aged 37. She comes in for emergency contraception, 60 hours after a split condom. She is very anxious, as this episode of sexual intercourse was not with her husband, who has had a vasectomy. It is critical he should not find out: they have two teenage children and she does not want to hurt either them or him. However, she also feels she could not give up her lover and therefore needs long-term contraception, in addition to her immediate need. This accident has made her realize that condoms are not good enough.

During the course of the consultation, she mentions that her elder sister had a DVT when she was 35. When questioned more closely, she vaguely remembers that an aunt may also have had a DVT, but she cannot recall any other family history. She herself took the combined pill in her twenties, without any problems. Her husband had the vasectomy because they felt their family was complete and she had been getting headaches which she felt were made worse by the pill. She is a non-smoker.

Our discussion first concentrates on the immediate issue of her need for emergency contraception. Although it would have been possible to give her PC4, it seems sensible to give her the progestogen-only method.

In the long term, I suggest a thrombophilia screen. However, Margaret is not keen. She would need to go to the hospital: 'How could I explain all that to my husband?' she asks, 'It's all too complicated.' She therefore decides she will simply find an alternative to the combined pill, as it seems sensible not to take unnecessary risks.

The next problem is that her husband has to be unaware of the method. This rules out IUDs (unless the threads were cut off and she doesn't like the uncertainty this would bring). Implants are also impossible as they could be felt and possibly even seen. Her frequent time zone changes make the POP too difficult to attempt. Condoms have already failed her and she feels the diaphragm is too complex (how could she carry it around all the time?). In the end she opts for Depo-Provera, as the injection would leave no incriminating evidence and she would have the peace of mind of a very effective method which she does not have to worry about. I warn her about the possibility of menstrual disturbance, but she feels she can easily blame this on her flying.

In fact, she became amenorrhoeic after the second injection, which, in her job, she felt was a definite bonus.

References

Benagiano G (1998) Venous thromboembolism and the pill. Learning from the past, venous thromboembolism and the pill: an endless saga. *Human Reproduction* 13(5): 1115–16.

Bertina RM, Koeleman BP, Koster T et al. (1994) Mutation in blood coagulation factor V associated with resistance to activated protein C. *Nature* 369: 64–7.

Broome M, Macaulay O (1996) Consider the progestogen-only pill. *Br J Fam Plan* 22: 111.

de Bruijn SFTM, Stam J, Koopman MMW et al. (1998) Case–control study of risk of cerebral sinus thrombosis in oral contraceptive users who are carriers of hereditary prothrombotic conditions. *Br Med J* 316: 589–92.

Campbell B (1996) Thrombosis, phlebitis and varicose veins. *Br Med J* 312: 198–9.

Clinical and Scientific Committee of the Faculty of Family Planning and Reproductive Health Care (1995) *Risk of Venous Thromboembolism and the Combined Oral Contraceptive Pill.* December. London.

Cohen J (1998) Recommendations on the safety of oral contraceptives are too important for the regulating agencies alone. *Human Reproduction* 13(5): 1116–17.

Committee on Safety of Medicines (1995) *Combined Oral Contraceptives and Thromboembolism.* London: CSM 1995.

CPMP (1996) *Position Statement on Oral Contraceptives containing Desogestrel or Gestodene.* April, 374/96.

Davies GC, Newton JR (1991) Subdermal contraceptive implants—a review: with special reference to Norplant. *Br J Fam Plan* 17: 4–8.

Department of Health (1996) *Oral Contraceptives—Clearer Information for Woman and Health Professionals.* Press Release, April, London.

Dunn N, Thorogood M, Faragher B et al. (1999) Oral contraceptives and myocardial infarction: results of the MICA case-control study. *Br Med J* 318: 1579–84.

Edwards RG, Beard HK, Bradshaw JP (1997) Balancing risks and benefits of oral contraception (editorial). *Human Reproduction* 12(11): 2339–40.

Egberg N, van Beek A, Gunnervik C et al. (1998) Effects on the hemostatic system and liver function in relation to Implanon and Norplant. A prospective randomized clinical trial. *Contraception* 58: 93–8.

Farmer RDT, Lawrenson RA, Thompson CR et al. (1997) Population-based study of risk of venous thromboembolism associated with various oral contraceptives. *Lancet* 349: 83–8.

Farmer RDT, Lawrenson RA, Todd JC et al. (2000) A comparison of the risks of venous thromboembolic disease in association with different combined oral contraceptives. *Br J Clin Pharmacol* (in press).

Fotherby K (1989a) The progestogen-only pill and thrombosis. *Br J Fam Plan* 15: 83–5.

Fotherby K (1989b) The progestogen-only pill. In: Filshie M, Guillebaud J, eds. *Contraception: Science and Practice.* London: Butterworth. 94–108.

Gerstman BB, Piper JM, Tomita DK et al. (1991) Oral contraceptive estrogen dose and the risk of deep venous thromboembolic disease. *Am J Epidemiol* 133: 32–7.

Greer IA (1999) Thrombosis in pregnancy: maternal and fetal issues. *Lancet* 353: 1258–65.

Guillebaud J (1989) Practical prescribing of the combined oral contraceptive pill. In: Filshie M, Guillebaud J eds. *Contraception: Science and Practice.* London: Butterworth. 69–94

Guillebaud J (1995) Advising women on which pill to take. *Br Med J* 331: 1111–12.

Hampton KK, Preston FE (1997) Bleeding disorders, thrombosis and anticoagulation. *Br Med J* 314: 1026–29.

Inman WH, Vessey MP, Westerholm B et al. (1970) Thromboembolic disease and the steroidal content of oral contraceptives: a report to the Committee on Safety of Drugs. *Br Med J* **2**: 203–9.

International Working Group on Enhancing Patient Compliance and oral Contraceptive Efficacy (1993) *Consensus Statement. Br J Fam Plan* **18**: 126–9.

Jick H, Jick S, Gurewich V et al. (1995) Risk of idiopathic cardiovascular death and non-fatal venous thromboembolism in women using oral contraceptives with differing progestogen components. *Lancet* **346**: 1589–93.

Laffan M, Tuddenham E (1998) Assessing thrombotic risk. *Br Med J* **317**: 520–3.

Lande RE (1995) New era for injectables. *Population Reports* series K(5): 23.

Le Blanc ES, Laws A (1999) Benefits and risks of third generation oral contraceptives. *J Gen Intern Med* **14**: 625–32.

Lidegaard O, Edstrom B, Kreiner S (1998) Oral contraceptives and venous thromboembolism: A case control study. *Contraception* **57**: 291–301.

Lewis MA, Spitzer WO, Heinemann LAJ et al. (1997) Lowered risk of dying of heart attack with third generation pill may offset risk of dying of thromboembolism. *Br Med J* **515**: 679–80.

Luukkainen T (1991) The levonorgestrel-releasing intrauterine device. *Ann NY Acad Sci* **626**: 43–9.

Machin SJ, Mackie IJ, Guillebaud J (1995) Factor V Leiden mutation, venous thromboembolism and combined oral contraceptive usage. *Br J Fam Plan* **21**: 13–14.

Martinelli I, Sacchi E, Landi G et al. (1998) High risk of cerebral–vein thrombosis in carriers of the prothrombin–gene mutation and in users of oral contraceptives. *N Engl J Med* **338**: 1793–7.

Medicines Control Agency (1999) Combined oral contraceptives containing desogestrel or gestodene and the risk of venous thromboembolism. *Current Problems in Pharmacovigilance*, Volume 25, June.

Mills A, Wilkinson C, Fotherby K. (1998) Can a change in screening and prescribing practice reduce the risk of venous thromboembolism in women taking the combined oral contraceptive pill? *Br J Fam Plan* **23**: 112–15.

Mills A, Edwards IR (1999) Venous thromboembolism and the pill. The combined oral contraceptive pill—are poor communication systems responsible for loss of confidence in this contraceptive method? *Human Reproduction* **14**(1): 7–10.

Poulter NR, Chang CL, Farley TMM et al. (1999) Effect on stroke of different progestagens in low estrogen dose oral contraceptives. *Lancet* **354**: 301–2.

Provan D, O'Shaughnessy DF (1999) Recent advances in haematology. *Br Med J* **318**: 991–994.

Redmond GP, Olson WH, Lippman JS, Kafrissen ME, Jones TM, Jorizzo JL (1997) Norgestimate and ethinyl estradiol in the treatment of acne vulgaris: a randomized, placebo-controlled trial. *Obstet Gynecol* **89**(4): 615–22.

Rosendaal FR (1999) Venous thrombosis: a multicausal disease. *Lancet* **353**: 1167–73.

Royal College of General Practitioners (1967) Oral contraception and thromboembolic disease. *J R Coll Gen Pract* **13**: 267–79.

Spitzer WO, Lewis MA, Heinemann LAJ, Thorogood M, MacRae KD on behalf of the Transnational Research Group on Oral Contraceptives and the Health of Young Women (1996). Third generation oral contraceptives and risk of venous thromboembolic disorders: an international case-control study. *Br Med J* **312**: 83–8.

Spitzer WO (1997) The 1995 pill scare revisited: anatomy of a non-epidemic. *Human Reproduction* **12**(11): 2347–57.

Spitzer WO (1998) Thromboembolism and the pill: the saga must end. *Human Reproduction* **13**: 1117–18.

Stadel BV (1981) Oral contraceptives and

cardiovascular disease. *N Engl J Med* **305**: 612–18.

Suissa S, Blais L, Spitzer W (1997) First time use of newer oral contraceptives and risk of venous thromboembolism. *Contraception* **56**: 141–6.

Szarewski A, Mansour D (1999) The 'pill scare': responses of authorities, doctors, and patients using oral contraception. *Human Reproduction Update* **5**: 627–32.

Vandenbroucke JP, van der Meer JM, Helmerhorst FM, Rosendaal FR (1996) Factor V Leiden: should we screen oral contraceptive users and pregnant women? *Br Med J* **313**: 1127–30.

Vessey MP, Doll R (1968) Investigation of relation between use of oral contraceptives and thromboembolic disease. *Br Med J* **2**: 199–205.

Vessey MP, Mant D, Smith A et al. (1986) Oral contraceptives and venous thromboembolism: findings in a large prospective study. *Br Med J* **292**: 526.

Vessey MP (1989) The Jeffcott Lecture, 1989. An overview of the benefits and risks of combined oral contraceptives. In: Mann RD, ed. *Oral Contraceptives and Breast Cancer: the Implications of the Present Findings for Informed Consent and Informed Choice.* New Jersey, USA: The Parthenon Publishing group, 121–35.

World Health Organisation Collaborative Study of Cardiovascular Disease and Steroid Hormone Contraception (1995) Effects of different progestogens in low oestrogen oral contraceptives on venous thromboembolism. *Lancet* **346**: 1582–8.

WHO Task Force on Postovulatory Methods of Fertility Regulation (1998) Randomised controlled trial of levonorgestrel versus the Yuzpe regimen of combined oral contraceptives for emergency contraception. *Lancet* **352**: 428–33.

Women at risk of arterial disease

Ian H Thorneycroft and Botros Rizk

4

Throughout this review women at risk for arterial disease will be defined as those at risk of myocardial infarction or cerebrovascular disease or accidents.

When selecting a form of contraception in patients with serious medical problems the risks of an unwanted or accidental pregnancy with this disease must be considered versus the risks of the contraceptive method.

Although the risks of the contraceptive may be high, the risks of pregnancy may be even higher

A poorly effective method of contraception, although less harmful to her disease process, may be more harmful for a patient when the effects of an unwanted pregnancy are factored in. Patients at risk of arterial disease have very high pregnancy complication rates and are the ones at risk of maternal mortality. A case from the literature illustrates this point:

'A 38-year-old woman who was diabetic and a heavy smoker and had incipient toxemia in a previous pregnancy came into a Planned Parenthood center in Little Rock, Arkansas, to renew her prescription for oral contraceptives (OCs). She was met with horror and told flatly that she could not use OCs. An intrauterine device (IUD) was too risky and tubal ligation was not acceptable, and she was told to use barrier methods. She did. She also became pregnant, developed toxemia, had a stroke, and her baby died. One may wonder whether an acceptable standard of medical judgment was exercised in advising contraceptives with a high failure rate to a woman in whom a pregnancy was potentially lethal to both mother and fetus. It might have been better medical practice to discuss in detail the benefits and risks of her various contraceptive options and let her make the ultimate decision, properly documented in the records' (Goldzieher 1994).

Deciding on the risks of a particular contraceptive method in patients with risk factors is complicated by the fact that few patients with risk factors are placed on combination oral contraceptives and consequently published studies have too few cases to analyse the interaction between risk factors and contraceptive use. Even when reported and analysed, the data are not presented in such a way to be helpful to the prescribing health care provider. What he or she wants to know is, 'Does a patient with a risk factor have a further increase in risk when prescribed a particular contraceptive?' To illustrate this point we note that study after study reports that patients with hypertension given combination oral contraceptives have an increased rate of stroke and myocardial infarction. For example, one excellent review of myocardial infarction and combination oral contraceptive (COC) use states that the Royal College of General Practitioners study reports a relative risk (RR) of 2.0 for myocardial infarction with COC use and a RR of 7.7 if the patient is hypertensive. The implication being that OCs have an adverse effect in hypertensives. Inspection of the publication by Croft and Hannaford, however, reveals that the RR of myocardial infarction in hypertensives prescribed COCs was virtually identical to those hypertensives not using COCs (Croft and Hannaford 1989; Petitti et al. 1998a).

Contraception for patients at risk of arterial disease

Strokes and myocardial infarctions are very rare events in women under 50 years old, and particularly under 35 years old (*Figure 1*).

Almost all stroke and myocardial infarction deaths in the UK and USA are after age 45 and 90% are after age 45 in Mexico.

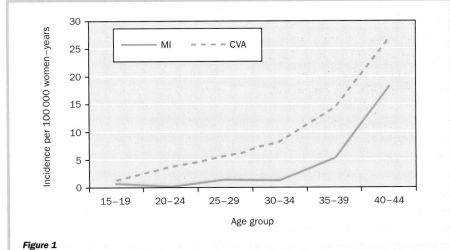

Figure 1
Incidence of myocardial infarction (MI) and cerebrovascular disease accidents (CDA), related to age.

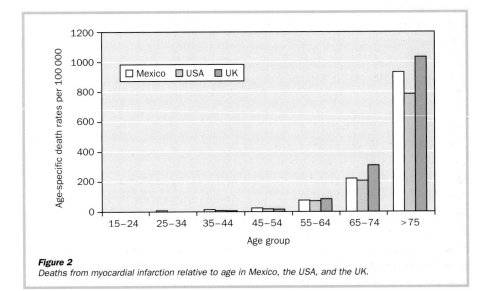

Figure 2
Deaths from myocardial infarction relative to age in Mexico, the USA, and the UK.

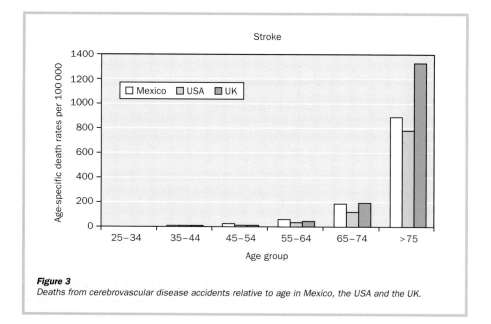

Figure 3
Deaths from cerebrovascular disease accidents relative to age in Mexico, the USA and the UK.

Most deaths from stroke and myocardial infarction are after age 45 years

If strokes and myocardial infarctions are increased by COC the attributable risk, that is the number increased by COCs, can only be one or two myocardial infarctions or strokes per 100 000 users (Petitti et al. 1997) (*Figures 2 and 3*).

Only hormonal contraception can potentially increase the probability of a myocardial infarction or a stroke and most attention has been placed on COCs. Barrier methods clearly would be safer, but with their high failure rate we do not recommend them, except in the most compliant patient. The complications of unplanned pregnancies can be substantial as was demonstrated in the clinical case presented above. We are also unfamiliar with any medical reason not to prescribe intrauterine contraceptive devices (IUCDs) to

Table 1
Key to abbreviations used in WHO recommendation tables

Type of contraceptive

COC	Combined oral contraceptives
CIC	Combined injectable contraceptives
POP	Progestogen only pills
NET-EN	Norethisterone (norethindrone) enanthate
DMPA	Depot medroxyprogesterone acetate
NOR	Norplant I and II implants
Cu-IUD	Copper-bearing intrauterine device
LNG-IUD	Levonorgestrel-releasing intrauterine device

Recommendation

I = Initiation
C = Continuation

1 A condition for which there is no restriction for the use of the contraceptive method.
2 A condition where the advantages of using the method generally outweigh the theoretical or proven risks.
3 A condition where the theoretical or proven risks usually outweigh the advantages of using the method.
4 A condition which represents an unacceptable health risk if the contraceptive method is used.

---

patients at risk of arterial disease, so these highly effective devices are probably the safest in these patients.

Throughout this chapter, reference will be made to the publication by the World Health Organization (1996) on *Improving Access to Quality Care and Family Planning: Medical Eligibility Criteria for Contraceptive Use*. Our discussion will on occasion be more liberal in condoning the use of some forms of contraception. The World Health Organization recommendations were reached after careful review of the literature. *Table 1* summarizes the abbreviations used in all the tables containing the World Health Organization recommendations.

Myocardial infarction

Major risk factors in women for myocardial infarction along with their relative risks, if known, are listed in *Table 2*. Genetic predisposition manifested by a strong family

Table 2
Risk factors and their relative risks for myocardial infarction in women

Risk factor	RR	References
Hypertension	4.7, 2.4	Sidney et al. 1996; Croft and Hannaford 1989
Toxemia	2.8	Croft and Hannaford 1989
Diabetes	17.5, 6.9	Sidney et al. 1996; Croft and Hannaford 1989
Lipids		
Elevated cholesterol	3.0	Sidney et al. 1996
Low HDL		
Elevated LDL		
Elevated triglycerides		
Elevated Lp(a)		
Smoking, current	8.3, 4.3	Croft and Hannaford 1989; Sidney et al. 1996
Truncal obesity		
Body mass, highest quartile	5.6	Sidney et al. 1996
Elevated plasma homocysteine		

history is also a strong risk factor. Many of these factors are interrelated such as lipids, diabetes, obesity and genetics.

All acute coronary syndromes (sudden cardiac death, all forms of angina, and myocardial infarction) result from instability of atherosclerotic plaques with intramural hemorrhage, fissuring, and plaque rupture, any one of which may precipitate acute thrombotic occlusion. Advanced lesions of atherosclerosis demonstrate (1) accumulation of intimal smooth muscle cells, together with variable numbers of accumulated macrophages and T-lymphocytes; (2) formation by the proliferated smooth muscle cells of large amounts of connective tissue matrix, including collagen, elastic fibers, and proteoglycans; and (3) accumulation of lipid, principally in the form of cholesterol esters and free cholesterol within the cells as well as in the surrounding connective tissues. Myocardial infarctions have been noted in 'clean' coronary arteries and may be a vasospastic and thrombotic phenomenon.

The relationship if any, between myocardial infarction and COC is quite confused in the medical literature. Early studies using high dose estrogen and progestogen pills reported an increased incidence (Mann and Inman 1975). These older high dose progestogen pills decreased high density lipoproteins (HDL),

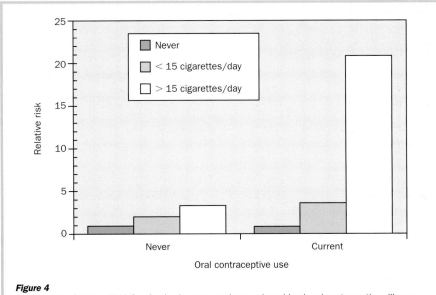

Figure 4
Relative risk of myocardial infarction in cigarette smokers and combined oral contraceptive pill users.

increased low density lipoproteins (LDL) and increased triglycerides. It was presumed, therefore, that these adverse lipid changes were the etiology of the increased rate of myocardial infarction in COC users and hence efforts were made to develop combinations with a lower progestogen and estrogen content, resulting in more favorable lipid profiles. Somewhat confusingly COC preparations which lowered HDL and raised LDL were found to decrease atherosclerotic plaque formation in monkeys. Stressed monkeys with very abnormal lipids and presumably at high risk of coronary disease had the most plaque reduction from OCs

(Adams et al. 1987a). This seeming paradox is explained by the fact that the estrogen in COCs is an antioxidant and prevents LDL cholesterol from being incorporated into the arterial wall (Ravi Subbiah et al. 1993).

Myocardial infarctions in women taking the pill are thrombotic not atherosclerotic (Bellinger 1993).

MI in pill-takers is thrombotic, not atherosclerotic

Past use of OCs is not associated with an increased risk of myocardial infarction, nor is the effect related to duration of use, which is further evidence that there is no effect on plaque formation (Stampfer et al. 1990).

From a theoretical aspect OCs should not increase myocardial infarction. Croft and Hannaford clearly demonstrated that when smokers were excluded, oral contraception did not increase myocardial infarction but that smokers who used COCs were at a higher risk than non-user smokers (*Figure 4*) (Croft and Hannaford 1989). The Transnational, WHO and Kaiser Permanente studies have also demonstrated no increase in myocardial infarction in patients given COCs who had no risk factors for myocardial infarction and in whom a blood pressure was taken before starting therapy (Lewis et al. 1997; Sidney et al. 1998; WHO Collaborative Study of Cardiovascular Disease and Steroid Hormone Contraception 1997).

COCs containing third generation progestogens may have a lower rate of myocardial infarction

COCs containing the third generation progestogens (gestodene, desogestrel and norgestimate) may have a lower rate of

myocardial infarction than COCs containing the second generation progestogens norethindrone (norethisterone) and levonorgestrel. However, these data need to be confirmed as the number of cases were so few and the data were not controlled for smoking (Lewis et al. 1997; WHO Collaborative Study of Cardiovascular Disease and Steroid Hormone Contraception 1997).

Progestogen only birth control pills (POP), progestogen only injectables, combined estrogen–progestogen injectables and Norplant® have not been shown to increase the rate of myocardial infarction (Petitti et al. 1998b; WHO Collaborative Study of Cardiovascular Disease and Steroid Hormone Contraception 1997; World Health Organization Collaborative Study of Cardiovascular Disease and Steroid Hormone Contraception 1998).

Cerebrovascular disease

A cerebrovascular accident is the infarction of central nervous system (CNS) tissue resulting from impairment of blood supply and oxygenation. Hemorrhage can result from the rupture of CNS vessels. The risk factors for stroke in women along with some known relative risks are listed in *Table 3*.

Pathologically strokes fall into three major categories: thrombotic, embolic and hemorrhagic.

Table 3
Risk factors for stroke

Risk factor	Adjusted OR (95% CI)	Reference
Smoking		
Non-smoker	1.0	
1–14 cigarettes/day	2.1 (1.5–2.0)	
>15 cigarettes/day	2.5 (1.7–3.7)	Hannaford et al. 1994
History of hypertension	2.8 (1.8–4.2)	
History of toxemia	1.4 (0.9–2.2)	Hannaford et al. 1994
Diabetes	5.4 (P < 0.001)	Lidegaard and Kreiner 1998
Earlier thrombolic disease	5.3 (P < 0.001)	Lidegaard and Kreiner 1998
Pregnancy	1.3 (NS)	Lidegaard and Kreiner 1998

Thrombotic

The majority are due to atherosclerosis, with the carotid bifurcation, the origin of the middle cerebral artery and the end of the basilar artery being the most common sites. Diabetes and hypertension are commonly associated with these kinds of stroke.

Embolic

Cardiac mural thrombi are the most common with myocardial infarction, valvular disease and atrial fibrillation being the most important etiologic factors for the formation of the thrombus.

Thromboemboli arising most commonly over plaques within the carotid arteries are also very important etiologic factors. The clots most frequently lodge in the distribution of the middle cerebral artery, where blood vessels branch and at areas of pre-existing luminal stenosis.

Hemorrhage

Intracerebral (intraparenchymal) hemorrhage: rupture of a small intraparenchymal vessel. Hypertension is the most common cause.

Subarachnoid hemorrhage

The most frequent cause of clinically significant subarachnoid hemorrhage is rupture of a berry aneurysm. Smoking and hypertension are predisposing factors for the development of berry aneurysms. Rupture is most likely after acute increases in intracranial pressure. (Such as with straining with defecation or orgasm.) Extension of traumatic hematomas, rupture of a hypertensive intracerebral hemorrhage into the ventricular system, vascular malformations, hematologic disturbance and tumors are also associated with subarachnoid hemorrhage.

Influence of contraceptive methods on the risk of stroke

COCs, particularly modern low dose ones, do not increase atherosclerosis or induce significant blood pressure changes or probably the risk of thrombosis on a plaque, and it is therefore difficult to imagine how they can increase the risk of stroke (Adams et al. 1987; Bellinger 1998; Cardoso et al. 1997; Halbe et al. 1998; Hite et al. 1999). However, COCs increase the risk of venous thrombosis and could certainly increase the number of strokes secondary to venous thrombosis. Patients who experience significant blood pressure increases on COCs could experience increased risk of stroke.

The literature on COCs and stroke is inconsistent. Reports frequently combine all varieties of strokes together or just consider one type. Many articles also combine fatal and non-fatal events and some even include TIAs (transient ischemic attacks). It is unlikely that if COCs do increase stroke, they would increase all types. A greater incidence of stroke has fairly consistently been reported for 50 μg

versus less than 50 μg COCs (*Table 4*) (Hannaford et al. 1994). Lidegaard has shown a decrease with decreasing dose, however 20 μg estrogen pills were virtually identical to 30–40 μg pills. Unfortunately, high dose estrogen COCs also contained higher doses of progestogen, which complicates interpretation further.

Modern low dose COCs do not increase the risk of any kind of stroke in healthy non-smokers

There also have been no differences demonstrated between preparations containing second or third generation progestogens (Heinemann et al. 1998; Lidegaard and Kreiner 1998). Most of the excess strokes previously reported may be explained by smoking (Hannaford et al. 1994). POP, injectable progestogen only, injectable estrogen–progestogen injectables and Norplant® do not increase the risk of stroke (Petitti et al. 1998b).

Table 4
Odds ratio of first-ever stroke by estrogen content of oral contraceptive used when event occurred

	Adjusted OR (95% CI)	
Dose of estrogen	**WHO**	**Lidegaard**
Mestranol or EE		
>50 µg	5.8 (1.5–22.8)	
50 µg	2.9 (1.7–5.0)	
<50 µg	0.6 (0.1–2.9)	
50 µg		2.65 (1.11–6.34)
30–40 µg		1.60 (1.05–2.43)
20 µg		1.59 (0.57–4.48)

CI indicates confidence interval; EE, ethinyl estradiol. Data taken from Hannaford et al. 1994 and Lidegaard and Kreiner 1998.

Contraception for patients with specific risk factors for myocardial infarction and stroke

It is our philosophy not to prescribe COCs to patients with several risk factors for stroke or myocardial infarction as their baseline risk is too high. These patients in our view are better treated with IUCDs, depot medroxyprogesterone acetate or sterilization.

Hypertension

Hypertension is a risk factor for stroke and myocardial infarction and by itself increases the risk of stroke 3–10 fold and myocardial infarction 5 fold (see *Tables 1* and *2*). The literature is not consistent in addressing this risk factor, although usually it is stated that patients with hypertension (or those in whom a blood pressure was not taken) prior to prescribing COCs have an increased risk of stroke and MI (Lewis et al. 1997; WHO Collaborative Study of Cardiovascular Disease and Steroid Hormone Contraception 1997).

The number of hypertensive subjects given any hormonal contraceptive is small and this is particularly true for COCs and therefore conclusions regarding the use of COCs are very difficult in this population. POPs are given much more frequently to hypertensive patients (WHO Collaborative Study of Cardiovascular Disease and Steroid Hormone Contraception 1998).

Table 5
Effect of COCs on the incidence of stroke in hypertensive patients

| | Adjusted OR – (95% CI for adjusted OR) | | Type of stroke |
	Non-users	Users	
Hypertension			
Transnational study (Heinemann et al. 1998)		*1	Thromboembolic
WHO 1998	4.94 (2.98–8.19)	10.3 (3.27–32.3)	Hemorrhagic
RCGP study (Hannaford et al. 1994)	4.8 (2.4–9.4)		All
Pregnancy induced hypertension/ toxemia (PIH)			
(Heinemann et al. 1998)		*2	Thromboembolic

*1 Users with and without hypertension showed no difference in stroke risk
*2 Users with and without PIH showed no difference in stroke risk

Table 6
Myocardial infarction: interaction of COCs and hypertension and toxemia of pregnancy

	COC use		
	Never	Former	Current
History of hypertension			
Croft and Hannaford (1989)			
No	1.0	1.5 (0.9–2.4)	2.0 (1.1–3.9)
Yes	5.4 (2.6–11.2)*	2.6 (1.3–5.0)	7.7 (1.2–49.2)
WHO (1997)—European Data			
No	1.0		3.85 (1.88–7.89)
Yes	5.43 (2.39–12.4)		68.1 (6.18–751)
History of toxemia of pregnancy			
Croft and Hannaford (1989)			
No	1.0	1.3 (0.8–2.0)	2.0 (1.0–4.0)
Yes	2.6 (1.3–4.9)	4.0 (1.9–8.8)	3.2 (1.0–10.9)
WHO 1997			
No	1.0		4.49 (2.19–9.2)
Yes	0.99 (0.45–2.19)		10.0 (2.4–42)

*Relative risk or odds ratio with the 95% confidence interval in parentheses.

Table 5 summarizes articles which have addressed the issue of whether or not COCs further increase the risk of stroke in hypertensive patients. The WHO study demonstrated an additive effect but the confidence limits are very wide. An unadjusted odds ratio calculated by the authors for hypertensive users versus hypertensive non-users was 1.85 (95% CI: 0.53–6.7), which is not significant and has a wide confidence interval. The other two studies showed no increase in stroke in users versus non-users. The risk of stroke appears to be greater for hypertensives given POP versus non-contraceptors; however, the confidence intervals are also wide and a crude odds ratio (OR) calculated by us was 1.24 (95% CI: 0.62–2.53) which is not significant. Estrogen–progestogen injectables had the same rate as non-contraceptors (WHO Collaborative Study of Cardiovascular Disease and Steroid Hormone Contraception 1998).

Table 6 summarizes the interaction of COCs and hypertension and myocardial infarction. Croft and Hannaford (1989) were unable to

Table 7
WHO hypertension recommendations.

Essential hypertension	COC		CIC	POP	NET-EN DMPA	NOR	Cu-IUD	LNG-IUD
	I	c						
a) **History of hypertension** where blood pressure cannot be evaluated (excluding hypertension in pregnancy)	3	3	3	2	2	2	1	2
b) **Blood pressure levels** (Properly taken measures)								
(i) 140–159/90–99	2/3(*)	2/3(*)	2	1	2	1	1	1
(ii) 160–179/100–109	3/4	4	3	1	2	1	1	1
(iii) 180+/110+	4	4	4	2	3	2	1	2
c) **Vascular disease**	4	4	4	2	3	2	1	2

(*) If blood pressure can be monitored periodically, then this situation is a category 2; if not, then it is a category 3.

demonstrate an increased risk of myocardial infarction in pill users over the hypertensive risk itself. The WHO study, however, did find an increased risk of myocardial infarction in hypertensive patients who were current users versus hypertensives who were non-users (*Table 7*) (WHO Collaborative Study of Cardiovascular Disease and Steroid Hormone Contraception 1997) although the confidence limits in the latter study were wide. Petitti in her review states that data from the Transnational study communicated to her showed no increase in myocardial infarction in pill users with hypertension versus non-user hypertensives (Petitti et al. 1998a; WHO Collaborative Study of Cardiovascular Disease and Steroid Hormone Contraception 1998).

Well controlled hypertensive patients can be given all forms of hormonal contraception

This is provided hypertension is their only risk factor and they have no existing vascular disease. They should be informed of their increased risk of stroke and myocardial infarction from hypertension and seek appropriate medical care to keep their blood pressure well regulated. As the stroke incidence has come down with decreasing estrogen dose, a 20 μg estrogen COC would be our recommendation in these patients. The WHO recommendations state that in well regulated hypertensives without vascular disease no method is contraindicated and an IUCD would be the safest method.

Diabetes

Diabetics have an increased risk of stroke and myocardial infarction (see *Tables 1* and *2*). As with the discussion of hypertension, COCs tend to be withheld from diabetics. In the WHO study the injectables and POPs were not however preferentially prescribed to diabetics (WHO Collaborative Study of Cardiovascular Disease and Steroid Hormone Contraception 1998). The authors can find no reports that address any increased risk of stroke or myocardial infarction in diabetics who are prescribed COCs versus those who are not. On the other hand it is difficult to find articles where sufficient diabetics have been given COCs to allow any firm conclusion. One report indicates no progression of nephropathy or retinopathy in diabetics given combination oral contraceptives (Garg et al. 1994). Modern low dose combined oral contraceptives raise both glucose and insulin so slightly that it is of no clinical significance. Glycosylated proteins and hemoglobin levels are also unchanged by COCs (Crook et al. 1993; Godsland et al. 1992; Kjos 1996; Korytkowski et al. 1995; Nader et al. 1997; Skouby et al. 1986; van der

Table 8
WHO diabetes recommendations

Diabetes	COC	CIC	POP	NET-EN DMPA	NOR	Cu-IUD	LNG-IUD
a) History of gestational disease	1	1	1	1	1	1	1
b) Non-vascular disease:							
non-insulin dependent	2	2	2	2	2	1	2
insulin dependent	2	2	2	2	2	1	2
c) Nephropathy/retinopathy/neuropathy	3/4	3/4	2	3	2	1	2
d) Other vascular disease of diabetes of >20 years' duration	3/4	3/4	2	3	2	1	2

Vange et al. 1987). The WHO is cautious about prescribing COCs to diabetics with nephropathy, retinopathy, vascular disease and diabetes for >20 years (*Table 8*). The authors agree and would only prescribe COCs to such patients when other methods are not accepted or feasible. Well controlled diabetics can be given low dose modern COCs and all other forms of hormonal contraceptives. They should be informed of their increased risk of stroke and myocardial infarction from diabetes and seek appropriate medical care and keep their diabetes well controlled. Again our preference would be for a 20 µg pill. Although the main problem with COCs and glucose tolerance has been the progestogen component, the lower dose of estrogen is recommended to theoretically reduce the risk of stroke. Troglitozone increases the metabolism of contraceptive steroids. Diabetics being treated with such agents should be placed on a higher dose COC and not a POP to avoid failure. IUCDs are probably also the best in this group. There has been one report of decreased efficacy of IUCDs in diabetics but this has not stood the test of time (Skouby et al. 1986).

Smoking

Smoking increases the risk of both stroke and myocardial infarction.

> *Those who use COCs and smoke have a 20 fold increase in the relative risk of myocardial infarction*

This increase is well above the relative risk of 3.3 for smoking alone (see *Figure 4*). COCs magnify the smoking risk even though by themselves they do not increase myocardial infarction (Croft and Hannaford 1989, WHO Collaborative Study of Cardiovascular Disease and Steroid Hormone Contraception 1997). It would appear that the major problem with strokes and myocardial infarction is also smoking (Rangemark et al. 1992). Prostacyclin does the opposite. Thromboxane is a strong vasoconstrictor and increases platelet aggregability and adhesiveness: it is increased in effect in smokers (Rangemark et al. 1992). Prostacyclin levels were not altered in smokers who were non-users of COCs, but were reduced in COC users who smoked. COC use alone also did not alter prostacyclin levels (Mileikowsky et al. 1988). Arterial thrombosis should be higher in smokers particularly those ingesting COCs.

Smokers under the age of 35 years and those who smoke less than 10–15 per day can probably be prescribed COCs as the incidence of stroke and myocardial infarction is so low. COCs should only be prescribed to smokers over age 35 under exceptional circumstances. A less pronounced effect on certain parameters of arterial thrombosis such as fibrinogen and fibrinopeptide A has been reported with 20 µg estrogen pills (Fruzzetti et al. 1994). Unfortunately, smokers have more breakthrough bleeding, and on that basis one would want to prescribe COCs with higher than 20 µg of estrogen (Rosenberg et al. 1996). Nevertheless we still recommend starting with a 20 µg estrogen pill. Other forms of hormonal contraception should be prescribed for women smokers over 35 years of age, except in very unusual circumstances and only when it is absolutely known that she smokes less than 10–15 per day. Any interaction between nicotine patches and gum, and myocardial infarction is unknown. Nicotine is vasospastic and it is probably best to treat such patients as smokers until more data are available. POPs and all injectables have unchanged myocardial infarction rates when compared with smoking non-users, the risk of stroke in these same smoking users was slightly elevated over smoking non-users although once again the confidence intervals were very wide. A crude OR calculated by the authors was 2.78 (95% CI: 0.91–856) for stroke when smoking users are compared to smoking non-users which is close to being significant. Many consider the POP to be a safer choice than COCs but these data would

not support this. Combined injectables had a lower myocardial infarction rate based on 1 case and 2 controls, the stroke rate was unchanged. IUCDs would be the safest choice in heavy smokers of any age and particularly those over the age of 35. *Table 9* outlines the WHO recommendations.

Thrombophilia

COCs increase venous thrombosis and are additive to the effects of the thrombophilias. Lidegaard did demonstrate increased risk of thrombotic stroke in patients with a history of thrombosis (Lidegaard 1993; Lidegaard 1997; Lidegaard and Kreiner 1998). Thrombophiliae are generally considered risk factors for stroke (Coull and Clark 1993). The probability of a thrombophilia increasing the risk of myocardial infarction is not well addressed in the literature, although it is stated as a risk for myocardial infarction in many textbooks. The incidence of factor V Leiden is somewhat elevated, but not statistically so in patients suffering an acute myocardial infarction with normal coronary arteries (Dacosta et al. 1998; Dunn et al. 1998; Holm et al. 1996; Manzar et al. 1997; Rosendaal et al. 1997; Siscovick et al. 1997).

The risk of increased risk of venous thromboembolic disease makes thrombophilias and previous thrombosis

Table 9
WHO smoking recommendations

Condition	COC	CIC	POP	NET-EN	DMPA	NOR	Cu-IUD	LNG-IUD
Smoking								
a) Age <35	2	2	1		1	1	1	1
b) Age >35								
light	3	2	1		1	1	1	1
heavy (>20 cigarettes/day)	4	3	1		1	1	1	1

absolute contraindications to COCs. We have no problems prescribing them to patients who are anti-coagulated to prevent ovarian hemorrhage at the time of ovulation and to prevent the congenital anomalies associated with warfarin.

Previous myocardial infarction

Most patients of child bearing age who have had a myocardial infarction are over 40 years old, a time of decreased fecundity. Only 10 of 158 myocardial infarctions were below age 35, and 25 of 158 below the age of 40 (Croft and Hannaford 1989). Physicians would generally advise against pregnancy and recommend sterilization except in the most rare of circumstances. Sterilization is probably best in this group; however, these patients do have a significant operative risk. The effects of COCs are unknown. A copper IUCD would appear to be the best non-operative choice. The risk of myocardial infarction in pregnancy for patients with a previous myocardial infarction is unknown. Badui reported that 18 patients thoroughly evaluated prior to conception, underwent pregnancy successfully. However, in the same review, two of five patients who suffered an acute myocardial infarction in pregnancy died (Badui and Enciso 1996). Patients with a previous myocardial infarction are thought to have a 10–15% mortality risk in pregnancy. It is impossible to estimate the risk in an unplanned pregnancy. *Table 10* summarizes the WHO conclusions.

Valvular disease and atrial fibrillation

There are no data. Patients who are anti-coagulated can probably safely take COCs and indeed this may be the preferred method to prevent massive ovarian hemorrhage and fetal anomalies from warfarin.

Patients who are anti-coagulated may have added benefits from COC use

In general COCs can be used safely in women with mitral valve prolapse without symptoms, other than anxiety. Otherwise, it would be prudent to use other forms of contraception. Antibiotic prophylaxis should be given before an IUCD insertion (Sullivan and Lobo 1993).

Increased intracranial pressure

An increased risk for stroke. There are no data available on the effects of any hormonal contraceptive agent. It is probably prudent to avoid hormonal contraception although pregnancy may be worse.

Table 10
WHO existing cardiovascular disease recommendations

Condition	COC	CIC	POP		NET-EN DMPA	NOR		Cu-IUD	LNG-IUD	
			I	*C*		*I*	*C*		*I*	*C*
Current and history of ischemic heart disease	4	4	2	3	3	2	3	1	2	3
Stroke (history of cerebrovascular accident)	4	4	2	3	3	2	3	1	2	2

Dyslipidemias

Low HDL and elevated LDL

The recent WHO study reported an increased rate of myocardial infarction for those with a history of abnormal lipids. It is not clear if the comparison was between dyslipidemia patients using and not using COCs (WHO Collaborative Study of Cardiovascular Disease and Steroid Hormone Contraception 1997). There are no other studies to our knowledge that have addressed this issue specifically. Modern low dose COCs, particularly the third generation, increase HDL and lower LDL. Monkey experiments reviewed above demonstrated that COCs decreased plaque formation, even when the preparation decreased HDL and elevated LDL. Furthermore, the monkeys with the worst LDL and HDL patterns benefited the most from plaque reduction by COCs (Adams et al. 1987). Guidelines suggested by Knopp for patients with elevated LDL cholesterol are illustrated in *Table 11* (Knopp et al. 1993).

The effects of depot medroxyprogesterone acetate and Norplant® on lipids are less well understood. Both slightly lower HDL and do not affect LDL. These agents would therefore appear safe in these individuals (Amatayakul 1979; Anwar et al. 1994; Garza Flores et al. 1991).

If a COC is prescribed then one with a favorable lipid profile such as a third generation progestogen containing preparation would be preferred, although not necessary. Such patients should be monitored and the contraceptive changed appropriately. The WHO recommendations are listed in *Table 12*.

Elevated triglycerides

An increased risk for myocardial infarction. Oral estrogens and COCs increase triglycerides. The triglycerides which are increased by estrogens are not athrogenic. A major concern is pancreatitis when triglyceride levels reach 1000 mg/dl (11.3 nmol/l). Baseline levels above 300–400 mg/dl (3.4–4.5 nmol/l) would be a contraindication to COCs. Norplant® and depot medroxyprogesterone acetate both slightly elevate triglycerides, but not to clinically significant levels (Amatayakul 1979; Anwar et al. 1994; Garza-Flores et al. 1991). No other form of contraception would be contraindicated in this circumstance.

Elevated Lp(a) and homocysteine levels

Estrogen reduces Lp(a); however, what few data there are with COCs are contradictory. Increased Lp(a) levels have been reported in COCs users; another report stated the levels

Table 11
WHO hyperlipidemia recommendations

Known hyperlipidaemias	COC	CIC	POP	NET-EN DMPA	NOR	Cu-IUD	LNG-IUD
Screening is NOT necessary for safe use of contraceptive methods							
a) Uncomplicated	2	2	1	1	1	1	1
b) Complicated (pulmonary hypertension, atrial fibrillation, history of sub-acute bacterial endocarditis)	4	4	1	1	1	2	2

Table 12
Recommendations for COC use in patients with elevated LDL-cholesterol levels

	Age			
	<35 years old		**>35 years old**	
	Number of risk factors			
LDC-C mg/dl nmol/l	**0–1**	**>2**	**0–1**	**>2**
<130	Yes	Yes	Yes	Yes
130–160	Yes	Yes with diet	Yes with diet	No
160–190	Yes with diet	No	No	No
>190	No	No	No	No

Data taken from Knopp et al. (1993).

may be better in a desogestrel versus levonorgestrel containing COCs. The latter effect was only seen in non-smokers (Shaarawy et al. 1997; Porkka et al. 1995). Clearly we need more data in this area and at the present time it would be prudent to avoid COCs in patients with elevated Lp(a). Clinically this is not a problem as these values are generally unknown. If they are elevated then the use of COCs would probably not be indicated, as the patient would likely have a severe cardiac or lipid problem which resulted in the need for this test.

IUCDs would probably be the best choice until further data are available.

Truncal obesity

Obesity by itself is not a contraindication to the use of OCs or any other form of contraception. These patients may have other abnormalities already discussed such as diabetes and dyslipidemias.

Genetics

Like truncal obesity these patients are likely to have a dyslipidemia, but in its absence there is probably no contraindication to COCs.

Summary

Virtually all forms of contraception can probably safely be given to patients at risk for arterial disease. The greater the risk for stroke or myocardial infarction from her risk factors the more consideration should be given to sterilization procedures or IUCDs. The safest reversible procedures to patients at risk for arterial disease are IUCDs. They are effective in preventing pregnancy and have no metabolic effects. Barrier methods are generally not recommended except in the most compliant patients due to the fact that their failure rate, and the complications of pregnancy in such patients, is so high. COCs, although considered by some authorities to be contraindicated in patients at risk of stroke and myocardial infarctions, are not necessarily contraindicated and can certainly be given in appropriate patients with appropriate consent. In the USA physician decisions are unfortunately strongly influenced more by potential litigation than medical or scientific fact.

Case histories

Case 1

Wendy is a 36-year-old insulin dependent diabetic with a 4-year-old son, who admits to an active sex life with a number of partners. She attends for contraceptive follow up, having been prescribed the COC pill 6 months previously.

'The doctor said I could use anything apart from a coil as long as my blood pressure stays low,' she says.

She is found to have a blood pressure of 145 systolic and 95 diastolic. She talks of the last time when her blood pressure was raised, when she developed severe pre-eclampsia in her pregnancy. It also transpires that her pregnancy resulted from missing three of her pills. She is told that the risks of her developing a stroke are now increased and that she must stop her pill. A discussion about the different forms of depot progestogen methods results in her requesting Depo-Provera. Condom use is also discussed with her.

Case 2

Jackie is a 22-year-old mother of three who takes beta-blockers for hypertension. She has a strong family history of hypertension and several of her elderly female relatives have suffered a cerebrovascular disease accident.

'I take the pill but I'm worried about what I've read in this week's magazine in view of my family history,' she says.

Her blood pressure is between 135 and 140 systolic and 80 and 85 diastolic after several readings. She is therefore reassured that her blood pressure is no contraindication to COCs. However, she has not been screened for hyperlipidaemia and her total serum cholesterol turns out to be 7.5 nmol/l. At a subsequent visit she is advised to discontinue her pills and offered an IUCD, depot progestogens or a progestogen-only pill. She requests a copper IUCD.

References

Adams MR, Clarkson TB, Koritnik DR, Nash HA (1987) Contraceptive steroids and coronary artery atherosclerosis in cynomolgus macaques. *Fertil Steril* 47(6): 1010–18.

Amatayakul K (1979) The effects of depo-provera on carbohydrate, lipids and vitamin metabolism. *J Steroid Biochem* 11(1B): 475–81.

Anwar M, Soejono SK, Maruo T, Abdullah N (1994) Comparative assessment of the effects of subdermal levonorgestrel implant system and long acting progestogen injection method on lipid metabolism. *Asia–Oceania J Obstet Gynaecol* 20(1): 53–8.

Badui E, Enciso R (1996) Acute myocardial infarction during pregnancy and puerperium review. *Angiology* 47(8): 739–51.

Bellinger MF (1993) Subtotal de-epithelialization and partial concealment of the glans clitoris: a modification to improve the cosmetic results of feminizing genitoplasty. *J Urol* 150: 651–3.

Bellinger MF (1998) Oral contraceptives and

hormone replacement therapy do not increase the incidence of arterial thrombosis in a nonhuman primate model. *Arterioscle Thrombosis Vasc Biol* 18: 92–9.

Cardoso F, Polonia J, Santos A, Silva Carvalho J, Ferreira-de-Almeida J (1997) Low-dose oral contraceptives and 24-hour ambulatory blood pressure. *Int J Gynaecol Obstet* 59(3): 237–43.

Chasan-Taber L, Stampfer M (1998) Epidemiology of oral contraceptives and cardiovascular disease. *Ann Int Med* 128(6): 467–77.

Coull BM, Clark WM (1993) Abnormalities of hemostasis in ischemic stroke [Review]. *Med Clin N Am* 77(1): 77–94.

Croft P, Hannaford PC (1989) Risk factors for acute myocardial infarction in women: evidence from the Royal College of General Practitioners' oral contraception study. *Br Med J* 298: 165–8.

Crook D, Godsland IF, Worthington M et al. (1993) A comparative metabolic study of two low-estrogen-dose oral contraceptives containing desogestrel or gestodene progestogens. *Am J Obstet Gynecol* 169(5): 1183–9.

Dacosta A, Tardy-Poncet B, Isaaz K et al. (1998) Prevalence of factor V Leiden (APCR) and other inherited thrombophilias in young patients with myocardial infarction and normal coronary arteries. *Heart* 80(4): 338–40.

Dunn ST, Roberts CR, Schechter E, Moore WE, Lee ET, Eichner JE (1998) Role of factor V Leiden mutation in patients with angiographically demonstrated coronary artery disease. *Thromb Res* 91(2): 91–9.

Fruzzetti F, Ricci C, Fioretti P (1994) Haemostasis profile in smoking and nonsmoking women taking low-dose oral contraceptives. *Contraception* 49: 579–92.

Garg SK, Chase P, Marshall G et al. (1994) Oral contraceptives and renal and retinal complications in young women with insulin-dependent diabetes mellitus. *JAMA* 271(14): 1099–102.

Garza-Flores J, De la Cruz DL, Valles de Bourges V (1991) Long-term effects of depot-medroxyprogesterone acetate on lipoprotein metabolism. *Contraception* 44(1): 61–71.

Godsland IF, Walton C, Felton C et al. (1992) Insulin resistance, secretion, and metabolism in users of oral contraceptives. *J Clin Endocrinol Metab* 74(1): 64–70.

Goldzieher J (1994) Cardiovascular disease in women. *Circulation* 68: 2941.

Halbe HW, de Melo NR, Bahamondes L et al. (1998) Efficacy and acceptability of two monophasic oral contraceptives containing ethinylestradiol and either desogestrel or gestodene. *Eur J Contracep Repro Health Care* 3(3): 113–20.

Hannaford PC, Croft PR, Kay CR (1994) Oral contraception and stroke evidence from the Royal College of General Practitioners' Oral Contraception Study. *Stroke* 25: 935–42.

Heinemann LAJ, Lewis MA, Spitzer WO et al. (1998) Thromboembolic stroke in young women. A European case-control study on oral contraceptives. *Contraception* 57: 29–37.

Hite RC, Bannemerschult R, Fox-Kuckenbecker P et al. (1999) Large observational trial of a new low-dose oral contraceptive containing 20 micrograms ethinylestradiol and 100 micrograms levonorgestrel (Miranova) in Germany. *Eur J Contracep Repro Health Care* 4(1): 7–13.

Holm J, Zoller B, Berntorp E et al. (1996) Prevalence of factor V gene mutation amongst myocardial infarction patients and healthy controls is higher in Sweden than in other countries. *J Int Med* 239(3): 221–6.

Kjos SL (1996) Contraception in diabetic women [Review]. *Obst Gynecol Clin N Am* 23(1): 243–58.

Knopp RH, LaRosa JC, Burkman Jr RT (1993) Contraception and dyslipidemia. *Am J Obstet Gynecol* 168: 1994–2005.

Korytkowski MT, Mokan M, Horwitz MJ et al. (1995) Metabolic effects of oral contraceptives in women with polycystic ovary syndrome. *J Clin Endocrinol Metab* 80(11): 3327–34.

Lewis MA, Heinemann LAJ, Spitzer WO et al. (1997) The use of oral contraceptives and the occurrence of acute myocardial infarction in young women. *Contraception* 56: 129–40.

Lidegaard O. (1993) Oral contraception and risk of a cerebral thromboembolic attack; results of a case-control study. *Br Med J* 306: 956–63.

Lidegaard O. (1997) Oral contraception and cerebral thromboembolism. *Acta Obstet Gynecol Scand Suppl* 164(76): 66–8.

Lidegaard O, Kreiner S (1988) Cerebral thrombosis and oral contraceptives. A case-control study. *Contraception* 57(5): 303–14.

Mann J, Inman W (1975) Oral contraceptives and death from myocardial infarction. *Br Med J* 2: 245–8.

Manzar KJ, Padder FA, Conrad AR et al. (1997) Acute myocardial infarction with normal coronary artery: a case report and review of literature [Review]. *Am J Med Sci* 314(5): 342–5.

Mileikowsky GN, Nadler JL, Huey F (1988) Evidence that smoking alters prostacyclin formation and platelet aggregation in women who use oral contraceptives. *Am J Obstet Gynecol* 159: 1547–52.

Nader S, Riad-Gabriel MG, Saad MF (1997) The effect of a desogestrel-containing oral contraceptive on glucose tolerance and leptin concentrations in hyperandrogenic women. *J Clin Endocrinol Metab* 82(9): 3074–7.

Petitti D, Sidney S, Quesenberry C et al. (1997) Incidence of stroke and myocardial infarction in women of reproductive age. *Stroke* 28(2): 280–3.

Petitti DB, Sidney S, Quesenberry CP (1998a) Oral contraceptive use and myocardial infarction. *Contraception* 57: 143–55.

Petitti DB, Siscovick DS, Sidney S et al. (1998b) Norplant implants and cardiovascular disease. *Contraception* 57(5): 361–2.

Porkka KV, Erkkola R, Taimela S et al. (1995) Influence of oral contraceptive use on lipoprotein (a) and other coronary heart disease risk factors. *Ann Med* 27(2): 193–8.

Rangemark C, Benthin G, Granstrom EF et al. (1992) Tobacco use and urinary excretion of thromboxane A$_2$ and prostacyclin metabolites in women stratified by age. *Circulation* 86: 1495–500.

Ravi Subbiah MT, Kessel B, Agrawal M et al. (1993) Antioxidant potential of specific estrogens on lipid peroxidation. *J Clin Endocrinol Metab* 77(4): 1095–7.

Rosenberg MJ, Waugh MS, Stevens CM (1996) Smoking and cycle control among oral contraceptive users. *Am J Obstet Gynecol* 174: 628–32.

Rosendaal FR, Siscovick DS, Schwartz SM et al. (1997) Factor V Leiden (resistance to activated protein C) increases the risk of myocardial infarction in young women [see comments]. *Blood* 89(8): 2817–21.

Shaarawy M, Nafea S, Abdel-Aziz O et al. (1997) The cardiovascular safety of triphasic contraceptive steroids. *Contraception* 56(3): 157–63.

Sidney S, Petitti D, Quesenberry C et al. (1996) Myocardial infarction in users of low dose oral contraceptives. *Obstet Gynecol* 88(6): 939–44.

Sidney S, Siscovick DS, Petitti DS et al. (1998) Myocardial infarction and use of low-dose oral contraceptives: a pooled analysis of 2 US studies. *Circulation* 98: 1058–63.

Siscovick DS, Schwartz SM, Rosendaal FR et al. (1997) Thrombosis in the young: effect of atherosclerotic risk factors on the risk of myocardial infarction associated with prothrombotic factors [Review]. *Thromb Haematol* 78(1): 7–12.

Skouby SO, Molsted-Pedersen L, Kuhl C (1986) Contraception in diabetic women. *Acta Endocrinol* 277: 125–9.

Stampfer MJ, Willett WC, Colditz GA et al. (1990) Past use of oral contraceptives and cardiovascular disease: a meta-analysis in the context of the Nurses' Health Study. *Am J Obstet Gynecol* 163: 285–91.

Sullivan JM, Lobo RA (1993) Considerations for contraception in women with cardiovascular disorders. *Am J Obstet Gynecol* 168: 2006–11.

van der Vange N, Kloosterboer HJ, Haspels AA (1987) Effect of seven low-dose combined oral contraceptive preparations on carbohydrate metabolism. *Am J Obstet Gynecol* 156(4): 918–22.

WHO (1996) *Improving Access to Quality Care in Family Planning: Medical Eligibility Criteria for Contraceptive Use.* Geneva: World Health Organization.

WHO Collaborative Study of Cardiovascular Disease and Steroid Hormone Contraception (1997) Acute myocardial infarction and combined oral contraceptives: results of an international multicentre case-control study. *Lancet* 349: 1202–9.

WHO Collaborative Study of Cardiovascular Disease and Steroid Hormone Contraception (1998) Cardiovascular disease and use of oral and injectable progestogen-only contraceptives and combined injectable contraceptives. Results of an international, multicenter, case-control study. *Contraception* 57(5): 315–24.

Women at risk of sexually transmitted infections

David Hicks

5

It must be remembered that unwanted pregnancy is not the only adverse event that can arise from heterosexual intercourse. Sexually transmitted infections (STIs) can be a risk for either partner and must be borne in mind by the family planning provider when helping to choose a method of contraception.

Perception of the need for protection from STIs usually emerges from a considerate and sympathetic sexual history, which should be elicited in a confidential environment. The contraceptive provider must be incisive and intuitive but respect social and cultural mores. A joint consultation with the sex partner can be invaluable. A comprehensive sexual history will permit the choice of contraception to be more appropriately made, and risk reduction may be suggested by changes in sexual lifestyle.

The potential interactions between any method of contraception used and STIs are not always considered by either user or provider. The user's risky behaviour may be ignored by both. A method could potentially put its user at increased risk of acquiring an STI, or conversely it might offer some protection.

Table 1
Factors influencing 'infectiousness' of STIs

Donor	Gender
	Genetics
	Genital ulcers
	Immunological status
	Intercurrent illness/infection
	Contraception
	Concurrent medication
Recipient	Gender
	Genetics
	Genital ulcers
	Immunological status
	Intercurrent illness/infection
	Contraception
	Concurrent medication
Organism	Size of inoculum
	Phenotype

Similarly, contraception might reduce the risk of transmission of an STI *from* its user or make it more likely. The clinical effects of STIs may be modified adversely or beneficially by contraception. Finally, any drug used to treat an infection or its sequelae may affect the contraceptive, and vice versa.

The clinical effects of sexually transmitted diseases may be modified adversely or beneficially by contraception

These interactions are only part of the complex equation between donor, recipient and organism which determines the 'infectivity' of STIs (*Table 1*).

To help the contraceptive provider, it is useful if we consider what is understood about some of the interactions noted above by looking at each contraceptive method in turn.

The male condom

The use of male condoms is promoted in most countries as the best non-behavioural protection against STIs, particularly human immunodeficiency virus (HIV), but we need also to consider its effectiveness in preventing pregnancy.

The efficacy of the male condom as a contraceptive differs according to such variables as age of the woman (and thereby her fertility), frequency of intercourse, quality of the product and experience of its users (remembering that it is a method designed for use by the male). With such variables operating and taking into account different designs of trial, it is perhaps not surprising that reported failure rates range from 4 to 23 pregnancies per 100 women in the first year of use. Analysis of publications up to 1994 suggests a failure rate of 3% annually with perfect use and 12% for typical use (Trussel 1994).

The problems of study design in trials looking at prevention of infection must also be understood. Allocation of any subject to a non-use or control arm, particularly where the infection studied may lead to infertility or even death, is ethically unacceptable. For condoms where spermicides are an integral part of the product, confounding effects are inevitable if the latter possess any antibacterial or antiviral property. Compliance may be uncertain. Trials of a prospective type are particularly difficult, but such concerns are being addressed (Macaluso et al. 1999).

The male condom provides greater protection against bacterial infections than against viruses

Scientific reviews suggest condoms confer high degrees of protection (reduction in risk to 50% and usually less) against STIs (Stone et al. 1986, Cates and Stone 1992, Hicks 1996). The protective effect, however, is usually measured for men. It appears stronger for bacterial than for viral organisms. There are three explanations for this. Firstly, studies in viral disease are fewer in number. This may be due to problems with study design related to the latent periods many viral infections exhibit, or perhaps because their diagnosis is more complicated. Secondly, viral infections such as herpes simplex or wart virus may be found on areas of genital skin not normally covered (and therefore protected) by the male condom. Thirdly, some infections may also be passed from non-genital skin and by contact which is not penetrative.

Women at risk of, or with, viral infections other than HIV are often advised to employ male condoms to prevent transmission, but there is a paucity of evidence from clinical studies to support this. In the same way, individuals treated for genital warts are often advised to use male condoms for, say,

3 months after the last lesion has disappeared. This advice, too, is empirical.

The risk of transmission of HIV in couples discordant for this virus has been extensively investigated (Lazzarin et al. 1991, De Vincenzi 1994), and such studies usually indicate an excellent risk reduction effect for this method, particularly in women. The latex condom is universally regarded as the 'gold standard' for preventing HIV transmission.

Condoms made of polyurethane are now available. These are undoubtedly stronger than their latex equivalent and thus should offer more protection against both pregnancy and STIs. Whilst technical information is available to demonstrate their strength, studies to show any enhanced protection against pregnancy and STIs are awaited.

Here then is a drug-free, safe, usually affordable, low-tech and non-prescription method of contraception which can also protect users and partners from bacterial and viral sexually transmitted infections and their sequelae. The question remains as to why the method is generally regarded as conferring relatively more protection from infection than it does against pregnancy, particularly since the latter has a period of maximal risk of several days either side of ovulation, whereas the former is a 'constant' threat. As stated earlier, the method is most effective with compliant male use. When being used to protect the wearer against infection, it may be used more compliantly than when used as an assurance against pregnancy for his female partner. Such considerations lead us to the conclusions that the user is as important as the method, and that patient selection and clear instructions on use and compliance are fundamental for success.

The female condom

Because the female condom is made of polyurethane and its outer ring covers the vulvar mucosa, it is to be expected that this condom is at least as effective as its male counterpart in the prevention of pregnancy, and perhaps more so in the prevention of STIs. A further advantage is that it can be inserted before sex by the woman and does not require the erect penis. In this way it may also protect by allowing the woman to avoid pre-ejaculate fluid.

Perfect users can expect a probability of contraceptive failure of 2.6% in 6 months of use (not significantly different from the diaphragm, sponge or cervical cap), with the same study estimating that such use can reduce the annual risk of HIV acquisition by more than 90% for women who have sexual intercourse twice weekly with an infected man (Trussel et al. 1994). There are no clinical trials in the area of this infection, however.

In vitro studies show that the intact polyurethane membrane is an effective barrier to viruses such as cytomegalovirus, HIV, herpes virus and hepatitis B virus as well as to gas and dye particles which are smaller in diameter than HIV (Drew et al. 1990, Voeller and Coulter 1991). The device has been shown to decrease the recurrence rate of *Trichomonas vaginalis* infection in previously diagnosed and treated women (Soper et al. 1993), and a Thai study shows that accessibility of the female condom can lead to a reduction in STIs in sex workers. The incidence of such infections was one-third lower than in those with access only to male condoms (Fontanet et al. 1989).

Some anatomical self-awareness and negotiation skills are needed for correct and compliant usage and cost may be an issue. Some studies report the frequency of the penis being misdirected outside the device or of the female condom being pushed into the vagina as problems, but these seem to respond to extra lubrication and practice. Loss of sensation and/or sexual stimulation can be less than with the male condom, but (for some) coitus using the female condom compared with the male version produces an increase in perceived sensation.

An effective barrier method that is not consistently and correctly used by high-risk populations cannot significantly interrupt the transmission of disease. However, a less efficacious barrier more frequently used can reduce the spread of infection. It is the poor acceptability of the female condom to women which has resulted in its full potential against STIs not yet being realized.

The female condom, therefore, has a place in the 'cafeteria' of contraceptive choice, but it needs commitment from the user and clear messages from the provider.

Other female barrier contraception

Reviews (Cates and Stone 1992) show that diaphragm or cap users have lower rates of bacterial and other STIs which can involve both upper and lower genital tracts. The risk of hospitalization for pelvic inflammatory disease (PID) may be more than halved for users compared with women using no contraception (Kelaghan et al. 1982). Since these methods are almost always used with additional spermicide it is difficult to estimate the protection provided by the barrier alone. On the other hand, individual women and some authorities (Stewart 1994) report that problems such as urinary tract infections, bacterial vaginosis, candidiasis and toxic shock syndrome may have an increased incidence in users of vaginal barrier methods. These methodologies do not, of course, protect the vagina and, whilst secretions from this organ contain a number of natural antibacterial and antiviral defence agents including lysosomes, polyamines, zinc, hydrogen peroxide and lactoferrin (Cohen 1991), protection against STIs cannot be assumed.

What is difficult to control for in studies of women-controlled barriers and infection is sexual behaviour. Women in such studies tend to be older, have more stable partnerships and change partners less frequently, and thus enjoy lower overall risk. The provider must enquire into such factors before advising these methods inappropriately.

Spermicides

There are a number of substances that in vitro are found to inactivate clinically important STIs including HIV. Nonoxynol 9 is perhaps the most researched and it has been shown to reduce the rate of gonococcal and chlamydial cervical infection (Kelly et al. 1985), but there are no clinical studies to date demonstrating unequivocally that spermicides prevent HIV infection in vivo.

On the debit side it should be realized that spermicides can cause vaginal mucosal erosions, irritation, reddening or ulcers, and that these effects appear to be related to frequency of use and dose. The clinical effect

is ill-defined and varies from the reporting of user complaints (often by sex workers) to researchers using colposcopic observations. Such 'inflammation' could theoretically facilitate entry for an STI.

A meta-analysis of published reports up to 1990 suggests that protection exists against *Treponema pallidum*, herpes simplex virus, *Chlamydia trachomatis, Neisseria gonorrhoeae* and *Trichomonas vaginalis*. The aggregated relative risk is 0.52 for 22 studies compared with an aggregated relative risk of 0.65 for 9 condom studies (Rosenburg et al. 1991). However, the largest randomized controlled trial of nonoxynol 9 film in around 1300 sex workers in Cameroon indicates that there is no additional protection for women in avoiding HIV, gonorrhoea or chlamydia beyond that offered by condoms alone (Roddy et al. 1998). Genital wart virus does not appear to be affected by nonoxynol 9.

For women using only spermicides for contraception, there is a risk of pregnancy of 6% after one year's perfect use, but 21% in typical use (Trussel 1994).

Researchers continue to investigate nonoxynol 9 and various formulations of other agents, since the idea of a user-controlled, effective, non-prescription, combined contraceptive-cum-microbicide which is cheap and safe has obvious potential worldwide.

Intrauterine devices

Intrauterine device (IUD) users can expect a 0.8% per annum risk of pregnancy, which is even smaller (0.1%) when the device contains progesterone (Trussel 1994).

Since the device acts as a foreign body and because there is no barrier to the cervix, there is concern about lower genital tract infections ascending to produce PID. Excellent reviews (Fairlie et al. 1992, Tcheng 1993) show us that the IUD itself does not introduce infection. It is the woman's (and/or her male partner's) sexual lifestyle and the presence or introduction of an STI that is mostly responsible for any increased risk of PID. Since most PID occurs in the first 20 days after insertion, and because the person who inserts the device (i.e. ideally, an experienced operator) is as important as the person into whom it is inserted, careful patient and doctor selection with scrupulous follow-up in the first 6 weeks is needed. Screening for STIs before insertion is also advised.

Intrauterine devices should only be inserted by experienced operators and scrupulous follow-up is required

The case for universal antibiotic prophylaxis at IUD insertion has not been proved. In women judged by self-reported medical history to be at low risk of an STI, indicators of acute or subacute pelvic infection (such as removal of the device within 90 days or access of medical services for gynaecological complaints), are no different in women given a placebo, when compared with others given a prophylactic antibiotic (Walsh et al. 1998).

Concerns about more frequent and more severe pelvic infection and IUD-related increased menstrual blood loss in HIV-infected women have led to suggestions that this method may be relatively contraindicated in such populations. A large study of about 150 infected and 500 non-infected Kenyan women showed no greater risk overall of IUD complications or infection-related problems in the former, regardless of the degree of immunosuppression, at 1 month and 4 months after insertion. The use of an IUD was found also not be associated with increased cervical shedding of HIV (Sinei et al. 1998). The method may be safely used by appropriately selected HIV-infected women who have access to medical services.

For healthy women judged not to be at increased risk of STI, the levonorgestrel-releasing IUD may actually reduce the risk of PID (Andersson et al. 1994).

IUD wearers with active viral disease (say, one of the hepatides) could experience increased menstrual loss and might, therefore, theoretically put any sexual partner at increased risk of transmission. Knowledge of the user's lifestyle and medical history is again invaluable.

Injectable contraception

For women using injectable contraception a theoretical increased risk of STI could arise owing to immunological changes induced by progestogens as well as by any subsequent chaotic menstrual loss. Reuse of non-sterilized needles and other equipment for administration might also be considered a transmission risk for viruses such as the hepatides or HIV. In practice, however, such risks remain theoretical, with no reported instances.

Women who use injectable contraceptives are, of course, included in populations studied for HIV transmission factors. A correlation has been shown with a relative risk of 3 (Rehle et al. 1992) but the sample size was small (77 women only). No published study addresses this relationship *a priori*. A relative risk of 0.5 for PID in users of injectable contraceptives (Gray 1985) may be accounted for by the increase in viscosity of cervical mucus. For women with active hepatitis B the World Health Organization suggests that injectable

progestogens are less desirable than other methods (WHO 1996). If this form of contraception is used, liver function tests should be regularly reviewed.

Protection from pregnancy is known to be excellent. Typical failure rates of 0.3% within the first year of use are noted (Trussel 1994).

Lactational amenorrhoea

It is disturbing to think that whilst the fully breastfeeding woman with HIV whose menses have not returned can rely on this as effective contraception for up to 6 months after giving birth, her chosen contraceptive method may place her infant at increased risk of infection. One in every seven children breastfed by HIV-positive mothers will become infected.

In the developing world the risk of death from malnutrition or infection through unclean water used in the preparation of milk-substitute formulas can be greater than the risk of HIV infection through breastfeeding. A balance must therefore be observed. The influence of this method upon the risk of transmission or acquisition of other STIs and their sequelae is unknown.

The method offers a less than 2% chance of pregnancy in the circumstances described above.

Sterilization

Female sterilization

Ligation or other surgical means of blockage of the fallopian tubes should protect the female upper genital tract from ascending pathogens but will have no influence on infection of the lower genital tract. The risk of PID should be reduced but any abandonment of barrier contraception might lead to a higher risk of lower genital tract infection.

Primary or recurrent pelvic inflammatory disease in sterilized women is reported. Transmission by fistulae or local lymphatic spread may account for these rare instances.

Women can expect a 0.4% risk of pregnancy per annum (Trussel 1994).

Male sterilization

In theory vasectomy eliminates sperm as a potential vector for HIV and other STIs. It has also been suggested that the inflammatory changes produced in the epididymis by surgical trauma might increase the number of infected leucocytes locally, such that viral entry into seminal fluid through accessory sexual organs is not prevented. The true situation for HIV or any other STI has not been researched.

What is known is that the method provides a 0.1% per annum risk of pregnancy in the female sexual partner (Trussel 1994).

Oral contraception

Many and diverse influences operate here and this methodology provides a good example of the complexities of the possible interactions between method, pathogen and other treatments.

It is probably easier to begin with the more certain expectation that a perfect user has of a 0.1% per annum contraceptive failure rate with the combined oral contraceptive (COC) and a 0.5% risk with perfect use of the progestogen-only pill (POP) (Trussel 1994).

Its lack of a barrier effect does not explain why, in respect to STIs, transmission risk appears increased for some organisms but for others the method appears to offer protection. For COC users risk seems to be increased for cervical *Chlamydia trachomatis* infection but for the same women there is a decreased risk of symptomatic PID caused by that organism (Wolner-Hanssen). This latter 'protective' effect does not extend to PID caused by *Neisseria gonorrhoeae*, however. The COC may be protective against symptomatic PID by causing inflammation to be masked at a tubal or endometrial level. Women with unrecognized endometritis are four times more likely than those with recognized endometritis to be COC users (Ness et al. 1997).

Use of the combined oral contraceptive pill may mask the symptoms of pelvic inflammatory disease

When we consider that unrecognized (and thus untreated) PID makes subsequent infertility more likely, and that untreated STIs are risk factors for HIV transmission, then we begin to see that these are subtle and complex but potentially significant interactions.

Bacterial vaginosis is found less frequently among women using COCs (Moi 1990) and so is vaginitis due to *Trichomonas vaginalis* (Roy 1991), but the jury is still out regarding candidiasis (Barbone et al. 1990).

For HIV infection, it is first worth reviewing the physiological changes influenced by the COC, which may influence STI risk. Regular and reduced withdrawal bleeds may limit the time available for transmission and also the amount of viral inoculum, and these factors could reduce the risk of a woman with HIV infecting her sexual partner. On the other hand, any breakthrough bleeding, bleeding

during coitus (perhaps due to increased cervical ectopy) and the weak immunosuppressive effect of oral contraceptive hormones could contribute to an increased risk of such infection. Increased shedding of HIV-1 genetic material from the cervices of women using COC has been observed. Viral shedding increased as the dose of oestrogen increased (Mostad et al. 1997). For a non-infected woman exposed to HIV sexually, the weak modification of lower genital tract immunity (principally mediated by oestrogen) may be a factor for increased risk of infection.

It is still not clear whether the COC or POP influences HIV transmission. Some studies suggest that women are protected (European Study Group 1981, Lazzarin et al. 1991), but others indicate that the risk is between 2 and 12 times greater (Plowde et al. 1992, Clementson et al 1993). A good review of all papers up to 1995 is equivocal (Taitel and Kafrissen 1995).

Many HIV-infected women will be in their fertile years and, wishing to avoid pregnancy, will use COC or a POP. Should they require also one or more of the drugs used to avoid or treat opportunistic infection, or have been prescribed antiretroviral therapy, it can be seen that drug–drug and drug–disease interactions must be considered. Some of these interactions are predictable or known. A classic case is rifampicin, which we can use as an example.

Rifampicin is an antitubercular agent and a prophylaxis for meningococcal meningitis. It is known to induce hepatic microsomal enzymes (specifically isoenzyme cytochrome P450) and so increase the second-phase metabolism of synthetic oestrogen and progestogen. The effect is potent but widely variable between individuals and is known to persist for a variable period after completion of treatment. The efficacy of all hormonal contraception is severely compromised by the concurrent use of rifampicin.

Possible interactions between drug therapy and oral contraception should be carefully considered

Women using oral contraception, either COC or POP, who need a course of rifampicin treatment lasting more than 7 days, should be advised to choose another appropriate contraceptive method. Women using oral contraception of a combined or progestogen-only type who need to take a short prophylactic course of rifampicin (7 days or less) should be advised to take extra contraceptive precautions as soon as

rifampicin is started and to continue taking their pill. Any pill-free interval should be omitted while taking rifampicin and for 7 days after its last dose. Extra contraceptive precautions should be used while taking the drug and for the 4 weeks after the last dose.

The vast range of drugs and their potential interactions are beyond the scope of this discussion, but suffice it to say that some contraceptive drugs (e.g. ethinyloestradiol) will, through a facet of their metabolism (increased glucuronyl transferase levels), be expected to interfere with other medications (e.g. the antiretroviral protease inhibitors) used in the management of HIV which share the same metabolic pathways. Women taking protease inhibitors who use COCs containing ethinyloestradiol can expect a decrease in effectiveness of the latter such that an increase in dose or substitution with another contraceptive is advised.

Considering the number of potential drug interactions, particularly with the flood of novel antiretroviral products, it is to be expected that similar interactions will be seen more often. The provider must consider also the potential for use of non-prescription and recreational drugs.

The provider will require up-to-date and individualized information for the HIV positive contraceptive user. This can be obtained from written reviews (Piscitelli et al. 1996), but these will, by definition, be out of date when published. I would recommend three valuable alternative resources:

1. Specialist sites on the Internet: try http://www.liv.ac.uk/hivgroup. or http://www.eudra.org/humandocs/ humans/epar.htm.

2. The pharmaceutical company manufacturing the drug will often provide drug information by telephone or fax.

3. Specialist medical groups: members can access the Clinical Effectiveness Committee of the Faculty of Family Planning and Reproductive Health Care of the Royal College of Obstetricians and Gynaecologists, at 19 Cornwall Terrace, Regent's Park, London NW1 4QP, UK.

Combination contraception

The attraction of adding a good preventative against STIs in the form of a barrier method to a proven, efficient, non-barrier method for contraception is obvious. The method was popularized in Holland when it was feared that sole promotion of condom use in order to prevent HIV infection and STIs would jeopardize the low unwanted pregnancy and

abortion rates by causing the abandonment of more effective methods of contraception. The method was first advocated at an international conference in 1992 (Lunsen 1993). It should be remembered that any increase in efficacy of contraception or protection against STIs is difficult to measure and has not yet been reported. The male condom and oral contraception may not be the only effective combination; this means that there is an opportunity to tailor contraceptive technology to the individual woman and her partner's requirements.

Attitudes amongst users of the male condom and COC combination are encouraging, with most considering the method positive and feasible. Women tend to be more positive about the method than men, with condom use perceived as the main disadvantage (Rademakers et al. 1996).

Conclusion

Sexual intercourse has inherent dangers and sexual abstinence is the only certain way of avoiding its unwanted complications. The consistent and compliant use of a good-quality condom offers the best strategy for the prevention of sexually transmitted infection, including HIV, but the IUD and hormonal methods are superior for contraception.

Table 2
Methods and their effects

Method	Increased risk of STI?	Reduced risk of STI?
Male Condom	• Viruses may be introduced on outside of membrane • A belief in 'total' effectiveness may lead to acceptance of risk	• Protects the cervix and vagina • Viri/bacteriocidal effect of spermicide
Female Condom	• Acceptability	• Protects cervix, vagina and vulva • Avoidance of pre-ejaculate
Other Barriers	• No vaginal protection	• Protects cervix • Viri/bacteriocidal effect of spermicide
Spermicides	• Mucosal inflammation • Nonoxynol 9 not effective against HPV	• Viri/bacteriocidal effect
IUDs	• Foreign body effect • Increased menstrual loss • Irregular heavy blood loss	• Levonorgestrel IUD may reduce risk/severity of PID
Injectable contraception	• Immunological changes • Any re-use of needles	• Increase in viscosity of cervical mucus
Lactation amenorrhoea	• Viruses present in breast milk	
Female sterilization		• Organisms may have access to pelvis blocked
Male sterilization	• Inflammatory changes in epididymis	• Sperm abolished as vector for infection
Oral Hormonal Contraception	• Immunological changes • Masking of STIs may facilitate HIV • Increased size of ectopy • Concurrent medication if HIV positive	• Regularity of menses • Concurrent medication if HIV positive • Reduces inflammation of PID
Combination Contraception		• Adds a barrier

Consistent use of a good-quality condom is the best strategy for the prevention of sexually transmitted infection

Research is beginning to reveal the complex interactions between method, microbe and chemical moiety (*Table 2*). We must be careful not to discourage women from excellent methods of contraception because of unfounded fears about an increased risk of an STI (particularly HIV). Likewise, we must understand that a thorough knowledge of the user's sexual behaviour is a potent tool in the prescriber's armamentarium. Sex may not be inherently 'safe', but it can be made 'safer'.

Case histories

Case 1

Fiona is a 33-year-old business woman, married to Simon who travels extensively to the Far East for his employer. She is now aware that in the recent past he has frequented prostitutes on his visits overseas and this admission has caused marital strain. She is keen not to become pregnant and is happy with her

IUD. They have expressed a wish to continue their relationship.

Simon has recently developed genital warts. The couple have been advised that a joint consultation is required at the sexual health clinic. There, both are counselled of the risks of concomitant STIs including HIV infection. Both have a full infection screen for other STIs which proves negative. Simon has a negative HIV test, and Fiona defers her decision to be tested.

Fiona elects to continue with her IUD and to reduce risk of transmission of genital warts by also using a barrier method. She chooses to use male condoms. She decides to review their use when Simon has had a negative HIV test at 12 weeks post-risk or upon complete clearance of his warts (whichever is the later).

Case 2

Tracey is 26 years old, a sex worker and has been infected with HIV for 3 years. She is asymptomatic and not on any antiretroviral or other treatment for her viral condition. She is desperate to avoid pregnancy and is adamant that she will carry on 'working'.

Combined oral contraception is advised with the concomitant use of male condoms for both clients and her cohabiting male sex partner who is believed to be HIV negative.

She is counselled on these methods and advised that she must avoid intercurrent STIs as well as prevent the risks of their transmission to others. She is attracted by the idea of using female condoms for clients who decline male sheaths.

References

Andersson K, Odlind V, Rybo G (1994) Levonorgestrel-releasing and copper-releasing (Nova T) IUDs during 5 years of use: a randomised comparative trial. *Contraception* 49(1): 46.

Barbone F, Auten H, Louv WC (1990) A follow-up study of methods of contraception and sexual activity in rates of trichomoniasis candidiasis and bacterial vaginosis. *Am J Obstet Gynecol* 163: 510–14.

Cates W, Stone KM (1992) Family planning, STDs and contraceptive choice. A literature update. *Fam Plan Persp* 24: 75–84.

Clementson DA, Moss GB, Wilerford DM (1993) Detection of HIV DNA in cervical and vaginal secretions. *JAMA* 269: 2860–4.

Cohen MS (1991) Vaginal mucosal defences. In: *Vaginitis and Vaginosis*, pp 33–7. New York: Wiley-Liss.

De Vincenzi I (1994) A longitudinal study of human immunodeficiency virus transmission by heterosexual partners. *New Engl J Med* 331(6): 341–6.

Drew WL, Blair M, Miner RC, Conant M (1990) Evaluation of the virus permeability of a new condom for women. *Sex Transm Dis* 17: 110–12.

European Study Group (1981) Risk factors for the male to female transmission of HIV. *Br Med J* 298: 411–15.

Fairlie TMH, Rosenberg MJ, Roe P (1992) Intrauterine devices and pelvic inflammatory disease; an international perspective. *Lancet* 339: 785–8.

Fontanet AL, Saba J, Chandelying V (1989) Protection against sexually transmitted diseases by granting sex workers in Thailand the choice of using the male or female condom: results from a randomised controlled trial. *AIDS* 12(14): 1851–9.

Gray RH (1985) Reduced risk of pelvic inflammatory disease with injectable contraceptives. *Lancet* i: 46.

Hicks DA (1996) The risks and benefits of contraceptive methods regarding sexually transmitted infections. *Br J Fam Plan* 22(1): 34–6.

Kelaghan J, Rubin GL, Ory HL (1982) Barrier method contraception and PID. *JAMA* 248: 184–7.

Kelly JP, Reynolds RB, Stagno S (1985) In-vitro activity of the spermicide nonoxynol-9 against Chlamydia trachomatis. *Antimicrob Agent Chemother* 27: 760–2.

Lazzarin A, Saracco A, Musicco M, Nicolosi A (1991) Man to woman sexual transmission of the human immunodeficiency virus. *Arch Intern Med* 151: 2411–16.

Lunsen RHW, van (1993) Double Dutch but double message in prevention. In: *Proceedings of the Second Congress of the European Society of Contraception*, Athens, 1993, pp 73–6.

Macaluso M, Artz L, Kelaghan J, Austin H, Fleenor M (1990) A prospective study of barrier contraception for the prevention of sexually transmitted diseases. *Sex Transm Dis* **26:** 127–36.

Moi H (1990) Prevalence of bacterial vaginosis and its association with genital infection: inflammation and contraception methods in women attending STD and primary health clinics. *Int J STD AIDS* **1:** 86–94.

Mostad SB, Overbaugh J, DeVange DM (1997) Hormonal contraception, vitamin A deficiency and other risk factors for shedding of HIV I infected cells from the cervix and vagina. *Lancet* **350**(9082): 922–7.

Ness RB, Keder LM, Soper DE (1997) Oral contraception and the recognition of endometritis. *Am J Obstet Gynecol* **176**(3): 580–5.

Piscitelli SC, Flexner C, Minor JR, Polis MA, Masur H (1996) Drug interactions in patients infected with human immunodeficiency virus. *Clin Infect Dis* **23**(4): 685–93.

Plowde PJ, Plummer FA, Pepin J (1992) HIV I infection in women attending a STD clinic in Kenya. *J Infect Dis* **166:** 86–92.

Rademakers J, Coenders A, Dersjant-Roorda M, Helmerhorst FM (1996) A survey study of attitudes to and use of the 'Double Dutch' method among university students in the Netherlands. *Br J Fam Plan* **22:** 22–4.

Rehle T, Brinkmann UK, Siraprasin T (1992) Risk factors of HIV infection among female prostitutes in northeast Thailand. *Infection* **20:** 328–31.

Roddy RE, Zekeng L, Ryan KA et al. (1998) A controlled trial of nonoxynol-9 film to reduce male to female transmission of sexually transmitted diseases. *New Engl J Med* **339**(8): 504–10.

Rosenburg MJ, Hill HA, Friel PA (1991) Spermicides and condoms in the prevention

of STDs: a meta–analysis. Abstract C–22014. *Ninth International Meeting for STD Research*, Banff, Canada.

Roy S (1991) Non-barrier contraceptives and vaginitis and vaginosis. *Am J Obstet Gynecol* **165:** 1240–4.

Sinei SK, Morrison CS, Sekadde-Kigondu C (1998) Complications of use of intra uterine devices among HIV-I infected women. *Lancet* **351**(9111): 1238–41.

Soper DE, Shoupe D, Shangold GA et al. (1993) Prevention of vaginal trichomoniasis by compliant use of the female condom. *Sex Transm Dis* **20:** 137–9.

Stewart FS (1994) Vaginal barrier contraceptives and infection risk. In: Mouck CK, Cordero M, Gabelnick HL, Spieler JM, Rivera R (eds) *Barrier Contraceptives*, pp 105–22. New York: Wiley-Liss.

Stone KM, Grimes DA, Magder LS (1986) Personal protection and sexually transmitted diseases. *Am J Obstet Gynecol* **155:** 180–8.

Taitel HF, Kafrissen MD (1995) A review of oral contraceptive use and the risk of HIV infection. *Br J Fam Plan* **20:** 112–16.

Tcheng C (1993) What have we learnt from recent IUD studies? A researcher's perspective. *Contraception* **48:** 81–108.

Trussel J (1994) Contraceptive failure rates. In: Hatcher R (ed.) *Contraceptive Technology*, 17th edn, Irvington: 637–87.

Trussel J, Sturgen K, Strickler J, Dominik R (1994) Comparative contraceptive efficacy of the female condom and other barrier methods. *Fam Plan Perspect* **26:** 66–72.

Voeller B, Coulter SL (1991) Gas, dye and viral transport through polyurethane condoms. *JAMA* **266:** 2986–7.

Walsh T, Grimes D, Frezieres R (1998) Randomised control trial of prophylactic antibiotics before insertion of intra uterine devices. *Lancet* **351:** 1005–9.

WHO (1996) *Improving Access to Quality Care in Family Planning. Medical Eligibility Criteria for Contraceptive Use*. Geneva: World Health Organization.

Wolner-Hanssen P, Eschenback DA, Paavonen J (1990) Decreased risk of symptomatic chlamydial pelvic inflammatory disease associated with oral contraceptive use. *JAMA* 263(1): 54–9.

Perimenopausal women

Ailsa Gebbie

6

A perimenopausal woman often faces particular difficulty when considering her contraceptive choices. She may be uncertain as to when she has reached natural sterility and may be concerned about the risks and benefits of particular methods of contraception at her age. Psychosexual problems become increasingly common and the perimenopause is a time of peak incidence of menstrual dysfunction, which may well affect the choice of contraceptive. In addition, the perimenopause marks the onset in many women of menopausal symptoms and there may be a requirement to assess the risks and benefits of hormone replacement therapy (HRT).

Menstrual dysfunction may well affect the choice of contraceptive method in perimenopausal women

Older women and fertility

Conception rates

In women, fertility rates decrease with age, and begin to decline from age 35 years onwards. There is good evidence that it is primarily the quality of the oocytes rather than the ageing of the uterus that reduces fertility in older women, as assisted conception rates in women undergoing egg donation are similar regardless of the recipient's age.

Chromosomal abnormalities

With increasing maternal age, pregnancy outcome is poorer with increasing risk of chromosomal abnormalities, particularly Down's syndrome. The incidence of clinically recognizable miscarriage in women over 40 years old is around 30%

Termination of pregnancy

Women over 40 years old have the highest rate of therapeutic abortion per total pregnancy rate, with nearly 50% of pregnancies ending in termination. This implies a substantial proportion of pregnancies in older women are unplanned and unwanted, and cause a great deal of psychological and social distress for the women concerned and their families.

Coital frequency

Coital frequency is another significant factor that affects conception rates in older women. Studies have shown that coital frequency is strongly and inversely associated with age, and women aged 40 years have intercourse on average half as often as women aged 20 years. However, with increasingly high divorce rates, many women in this age group may be entering new relationships with a corresponding increase in sexual activity.

Hormonal changes and menstrual patterns

A woman's last spontaneous menstrual period occurs on average at the age of 51 years and is obviously a diagnosis made in retrospect. *Figure 1* illustrates the menstrual changes at the end of reproductive life.

The postmenopausal period is characterized by very low oestrogen levels and elevated gonadotrophin levels. During the perimenopause, oestrogen and gonadotrophin levels vary markedly and are rarely of value in predicting when contraception can be discontinued. An isolated measurement of elevated follicle-stimulating hormone (FSH) level is not indicative of total ovarian failure as subsequent ovulation may still occur.

In the years prior to the menopause declining

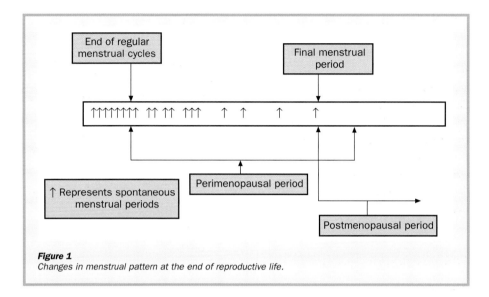

Figure 1
Changes in menstrual pattern at the end of reproductive life.

ovarian function can considerably disrupt the menstrual pattern, with increasing spells of anovulation, oligomenorrhoea and irregular bleeding. Many older women are referred for gynaecological investigation because of this, and pre-existing menstrual dysfunction significantly affects contraceptive choice.

When should contraception be stopped?

Contraception should be continued until complete natural sterility has been achieved and ovulation has ceased (*Figure 2*). The

oldest woman to give birth in the UK following a natural conception was 55 years old, although advances in assisted conception techniques have made pregnancies possible in postmenopausal women in their sixties using donor oocytes.

Contraception should be continued until complete natural sterility has been achieved

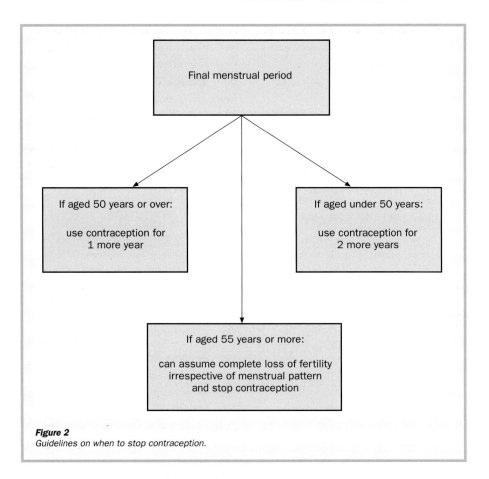

Figure 2
Guidelines on when to stop contraception.

Contraception in older women

There are striking changes in the pattern of contraceptive usage with age:

- Hormonal contraception is primarily used by young women in their teens and twenties despite major advantages in terms of reliability and gynaecological benefit for older women.

- Intrauterine devices are not popular in

the UK and are mainly used by women in their thirties. The hormone-releasing intrauterine system has been a useful addition to the range and has particular benefits for older women.

• Usage of condoms declines with age although they should always be recommended in new relationships irrespective of age.

• More than 50% of sexually active women who reach the menopause will be relying on either a male or female permanent method of contraception. More men and women are sterilized in the UK than in any other European country—a fact that reflects the difficulty individuals have in finding acceptable and safe methods of reversible contraception.

The use of condoms should be recommended in all new relationships regardless of age

Choice of contraceptive method
Combined oral contraceptive pill

The combined oral contraceptive (COC) pill is highly effective, safe and convenient, and has been studied more intensively than any other medication in history. It remains, however, a method primarily used by young women, and many women in the older reproductive years have undue concerns about its safety. There is no upper age limit to its use by healthy, low-risk, non-smoking women who, in practice, may continue with the COC until the age of 50 years. Women who smoke must still be advised to discontinue COC at the age of 35 years.

Gynaecological benefits
The COC has particular advantages for older women particularly with respect to menstrual problems, which become more common with age. It is a highly effective treatment for menorrhagia, premenstrual syndrome and dysmenorrhoea. The incidence of menstrual problems in women in their forties is high and carries large economic costs in terms of health care and absenteeism from work in otherwise healthy women (Coulter et al. 1995). Long-term COC users have a reduced incidence of diagnostic laparoscopy and curettage, and—more importantly—hysterectomy. Use of the COC indisputably lowers the risk of both endometrial and epithelial ovarian cancer by about 40–50%, although these benefits are frequently overlooked in any discussion of the risks and benefits of COC for older women (IPPF 1998).

Venous thromboembolism
It is well established that the COC is

associated with increased relative risk of venous thromboembolism (VTE). Risk of VTE increases with age and therefore particular caution should be taken when prescribing a COC to an older woman with any relative risk factors for VTE such as obesity, immobility, etc. Following evidence that use of third-generation progestogen-containing COCs had a slightly higher risk of VTE, the Committee on Safety of Medicines in the UK recommended that women should be prescribed the older, second-generation COC in preference to third-generation pills (Carnall 1995). This restriction has now been retracted, and the choice of COC for older women should be based on giving the lowest oestrogen dose that is adequate for good cycle control.

Cardiovascular disease

The incidence of cardiovascular disease with COC is now extremely small since low-dose pills are universally prescribed and women with significant risk factors rarely take COC. The incidences of both myocardial infarction and stroke have decreased generally in young women over the last 20–30 years. Reviewing all the available evidence, COC users who do not smoke, who have their blood pressure checked regularly and who do not have high blood pressure have no increased risk of myocardial infarction and little increased risk of stroke (Skegg 1999).

Breast cancer

The most comprehensive reanalysis of all the COC data and breast cancer was published in 1996 (Collaborative Group on Hormonal Factors in Breast Cancer 1996). Although generally reassuring overall, the small increase in relative risk of 1.24 found is of more significance to older COC users because the background incidence of breast cancer rises steeply between the ages 35 years and 50 years. Once the COC is discontinued, the excess risk of breast cancer declines progressively until disappearing after 10 years. Again, for older COC users this is of more concern as the increased risk after stopping COC will persist up to age 55 or 60 years. In practice, this slightly increased risk of breast cancer must not be viewed in isolation and is outweighed for most women in terms of effective contraception and non-contraceptive benefits.

Menopause

Use of COC in the older age group will mask the onset of the natural menopause. The COC will perpetuate regular withdrawal bleeds for as long as it is continued and will also treat any vasomotor symptoms and maintain bone mineral density. It can be used as an alternative to hormone replacement therapy, particularly in young women with a premature menopause, and the usual prescribing guidelines apply. The COC suppresses gonadotrophin levels and therefore there is no reliable hormone test that can be used to diagnose menopause in a COC user. When a women taking the COC reaches the age of 50 years, it should be discontinued and she should be advised to use the progestogen-only pill or a barrier method in the meantime. This will allow assessment of her current menstrual cycle and menopausal status, and thereby her requirements for contraception and hormone replacement therapy (*Figure 3*).

Progestogen-only methods

Progestogen-only pill

The progestogen-only pill (POP) is a highly effective and safe method of contraception for older women. Whilst the failure rate overall of POP is 2–3 per hundred woman years (HWY), among women over 40 years the rate is only 0.3 per HWY, which compares very favourably with the use of the COC in young women. The dose of progestogen in these pills is very low and it can be prescribed to women who smoke and have other risk factors for cardiovascular diseases and past venous thromboembolism. The major drawback of POP is menstrual irregularity, although amenorrhoea is a more common feature when older women take POP.

The POP does not suppress gonadotrophin secretion. In POP users over the age of 45 years with amenorrhoea, annual gonadotrophin levels can be undertaken to diagnose the onset of ovarian failure. In the presence of a raised FSH level, the POP should be continued for one further year.

Depot medroxyprogesterone acetate

Depot medroxyprogesterone acetate (DMPA, Depo-Provera) is an extremely effective method of contraception at all ages. It is a significantly higher-dose progestogen than POP and has more marked suppressive effect on gonadotrophin secretion and ovarian function. It will improve menstrual disturbances and can be particularly effective in treating premenstrual syndrome. Concerns exist, however, about its effect in the long term on bone mineral density and fracture risk in DMPA users with prolonged amenorrhoea (Cundy et al. 1991). It is probably prudent to discontinue the use of DMPA at around the age of 45 years to allow any loss of bone mineral density to recover prior to the onset of the menopause. Theoretically, systemic oestrogen can be prescribed in conjunction with DMPA for women deemed to be at increased risk, although in practice it is often simpler to stop the DMPA. Recent data confirm that DMPA and POP do not increase the risks of acute myocardial infarction, venous thromboembolism or stroke (WHO 1998).

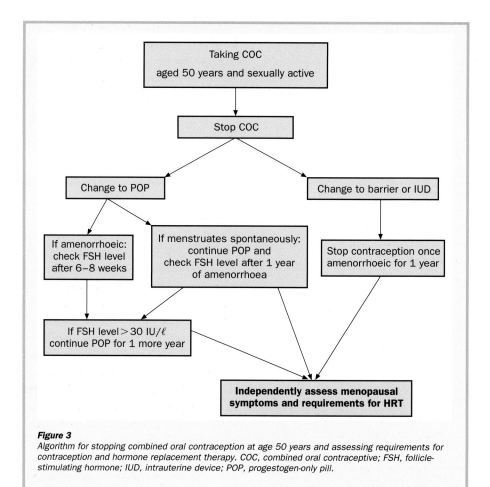

Figure 3
Algorithm for stopping combined oral contraception at age 50 years and assessing requirements for contraception and hormone replacement therapy. COC, combined oral contraceptive; FSH, follicle-stimulating hormone; IUD, intrauterine device; POP, progestogen-only pill.

Emergency contraception

There is no upper age limit to the use of hormonal emergency contraception if an older woman is judged to be at risk of pregnancy.

The usual contraindications apply, and if continuing contraception is required then fitting of an intrauterine device may be the method of choice.

There is no upper age limit to the use of hormonal emergency contraception

they may be the only methods acceptable to some couples, ovarian functions will be less predictable as women become perimenopausal and the signs of ovulation may be more difficult to interpret.

Barrier methods

Condoms should be recommended in new relationships at all ages for personal protection against sexually transmitted infections. Couples may find it difficult at older ages to initiate their use for the first time and they may exacerbate erectile difficulties. Women should be advised that the tensile strength of condoms can be drastically affected by oil-based lubricants and some antifungal preparations, leading to condoms splitting. Diaphragms have declined significantly in popularity since the 1970s but are relatively more popular among older women, many of whom may rarely consult health-care professionals. Uterovaginal prolapse may make secure fitting and retention of a diaphragm more difficult and use of a cervical cap may overcome this problem. Some older women appreciate the extra lubrication provided by the adjunctive spermicide when vaginal dryness is a problem.

Natural methods of family planning

Natural methods rely on periodic abstinence and fertility awareness techniques. Although

Intrauterine methods

There has been a resurgence of interest by women in intrauterine contraception with the introduction of the hormone-releasing intrauterine system and the adverse media coverage of recent COC data. Many women, however, are still reluctant to consider having an intrauterine device (IUD), despite the advantages of a highly effective, long-term method of contraception which requires no regular motivation other than the initial fitting. Older IUD users have lower rates of intrauterine and ectopic pregnancy, expulsion and infection. The risk of pelvic infection with an IUD is not increased in women of any age within a mutually monogamous relationship. As older women are more likely to be within a stable partnership, the IUD is a recommendable choice. The large, inert plastic devices are no longer manufactured but it is not uncommon to remove one from a menopausal woman after it has provided many years of effective contraception.

It is of prime importance to take into account an older woman's pre-existing menstrual pattern prior to fitting an IUD. Even the smallest copper-bearing IUD increases menstrual blood loss and pelvic pain, so a perimenopausal woman with significant pre-existing menstrual problems is not a good candidate for an IUD. Most IUDs remain effective far longer than the manufacturer's recommended 3–5 years, and when a copper-bearing IUD is fitted in a woman over the age of 40 years it can remain *in situ* until she becomes menopausal (Tacchi 1991). An IUD should be removed 1 year after the last spontaneous menstrual period. It is always recommended that an IUD be ultimately removed in a postmenopausal woman, as occasionally it can become a focus of major sepsis.

Levonorgestrel-releasing intrauterine system
The levonorgestrel-releasing intrauterine system (LNG IUS) offers particular health benefits for older women. The release of levonorgestrel into the endometrial cavity induces endometrial atrophy. Menstrual loss is significantly reduced and the LNG IUS offers a real alternative to hysterectomy in women with menorrhagia (Barrington and Bowen-Simpkins 1997). By the end of 1 year of use, around one in five women will be amenorrhoeic. Ovarian function is effectively unchanged and use of a LNG IUS does not alter onset of the menopause or menopausal symptoms. Although it is about ten times as expensive as a conventional IUD, its use can be justified as a cost-effective option in

selected women with menstrual dysfunction. The LNG IUS also has significant potential to provide the progestogen component of an HRT regimen in conjunction with systemic oestrogen (Raudaskoski et al. 1995) and therefore in many ways it could be the ideal method of contraception for the perimenopausal woman. The LNG IUS will not suit all women and minor side-effects occur frequently, particularly in the first few months of use. Women must have careful counselling about this prior to insertion to increase acceptability and continuation. The advantages and disadvantages of LNG IUS and how they relate to the older woman are summarized in **Table 1.**

The levonorgestrel IUS offers a real alternative to hysterectomy in women with menorrhagia

Sterilization

Sterilization procedures for both men and women increase in popularity with age, as older individuals become certain they no longer wish the option of parenthood. Uptake of sterilization is substantially higher in the UK than in many other European countries.

Table 1
Advantages and disadvantages of the levonorgestrel-releasing intrauterine system for the perimenopausal woman.

Advantages	Disadvantages
Contraceptive As effective as female sterilization Convenient, requiring no regular motivation	Many women dislike the idea of intrauterine insertion Insertion may be technically more difficult as the device is wider
Gynaecological Reduces menstrual blood loss Reduces dysmenorrhoea May improve PMS	Erratic bleeding and spotting in the first few months of use are very common Mild hormonal side-effects may occur such as acne, breast tenderness, nausea
HRT Has potential to be used as progestogen component of HRT regimen (although not currently licensed for this) Offers 'no period' HRT regimen	Erratic bleeding and spotting may occur when oestrogen is introduced

HRT, hormone replacement therapy; PMS, premenstrual syndrome.

Vasectomy is slightly more common in younger age groups; thereafter, female sterilization becomes more common. Common sense dictates that women who are near the menopause and require contraception for a relatively short period would wish to avoid undergoing an operative procedure. The existence of a post-tubal sterilization syndrome causing abnormal menstrual bleeding, pain and premenstrual syndrome has been questioned, although there is a noticeable trend of increased hysterectomy rates following sterilization. It is thought that women who are prepared to be surgically sterilized are more likely to seek a surgical solution to their menstrual problems and that changes in menstrual pattern following sterilization are primarily related to changes in contraceptive method (Gentile et al. 1998).

The menopause
Starting HRT

For many women, the perimenopause marks the onset of unpleasant vasomotor and psychological symptoms associated with the menopause. Women therefore will often commence an HRT preparation for symptomatic relief while still menstruating, either regularly or irregularly. As HRT will induce regular withdrawal bleeds, considerable confusion can arise regarding issues relating to fertility and contraception.

Practical prescribing points

- When HRT is initiated in perimenopausal women, it should be commenced within a few days of menstruation in order to obtain the best cycle control. Cheap, oral preparations are generally used in the first instance containing continuous oestrogen and 12–14 days of progestogen each month (sequential HRT).

- Perimenopausal women can use long-cyclic HRT, i.e. preparations giving a withdrawal bleed every 3 months. Women should be warned that erratic bleeding is common with these preparations.

- Hormone replacement therapy is not a method of contraception. The dose of natural oestrogen contained within standard HRT products is not potent enough to reliably inhibit ovulation. Adjunctive contraception must always be discussed with women who are not yet at

the end of natural fertility. There are numerous reports of women becoming pregnant while taking HRT.

- When sequential HRT is commenced in postmenopausal women, HRT withdrawal bleeds will occur. It is important to reassure women that these induced bleeds do not indicate the return of fertility. It is not necessary to restart contraception.

- The continuous combined 'no period' regimens are designed for postmenopausal women and are not recommended in the perimenopause. As a perimenopausal woman still has some endogenous ovarian activity, erratic bleeding will almost certainly occur and lead to confusion regarding the possibility of underlying gynaecological disease.

HRT and methods of contraception

Condoms, a diaphragm and an IUD can all be used in conjunction with HRT. The POP is recommended for use in combination with HRT and appears effective, although there are no scientific data to support its use in this situation. For simplicity, a sequential HRT preparation and POP should be given as two separate prescriptions. Most women find that they continue to have regular but scanty withdrawal bleeds with this combination. The LNG IUS can be used as part of an HRT regimen with systemic oestrogen only, although this combination is currently unlicensed.

Stopping contraception when taking HRT

As HRT masks the natural menstrual pattern, advising women on when to discontinue contraception while taking HRT is complex. The algorithm in *Figure 4* can be followed.

Case histories

Case 1

Dorothy is a 47-year-old dentist who has been married for many years and has teenage children. Recently she has begun to experience slightly heavy, but regular menstrual periods. She has been feeling a little low in her mood and wonders if she is beginning to notice some hot flushes. She is in excellent general health, exercises regularly and is slim. Over the years, she has mainly relied on a diaphragm and condoms for contraception. She attends her general practitioner asking for advice about her periods and whether she needs to continue contraception. She also asks if she could have a 'hormone test' for the menopause.

Dorothy's doctor examines her and finds the uterus to be of normal size. Dorothy has recently had a cervical smear that gave a normal result. The doctor explains that there is no need to measure any hormone levels, as the result would almost certainly not show any signs of the menopause and therefore may be falsely misleading. The doctor also explains that it is not uncommon to experience hot flushes while still having a regular menstrual cycle in a woman of her age and it probably represents early signs of the menopause. Although there is a natural decline in fertility with age, contraception is definitely still required, as it is likely that she is still ovulating.

As Dorothy is slim and fit with no risk factors for arterial disease, it would be appropriate to offer her the combined oral contraceptive pill. This would reduce her menstrual bleeding, give her excellent contraception and also treat any vasomotor symptoms. It could be continued until the age of 50 years. An alternative strategy would be to fit an intrauterine hormone-releasing system for contraception and to help reduce menstrual blood loss.

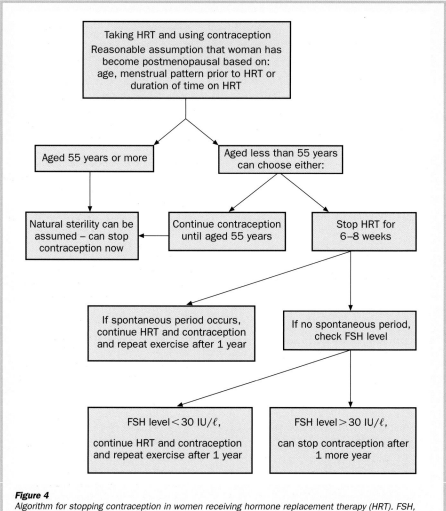

Figure 4
Algorithm for stopping contraception in women receiving hormone replacement therapy (HRT). FSH, follicle-stimulating hormone.

Case 2

Alison is a 51-year-old housewife who commenced hormone replacement therapy one year ago for hot flushes and mood swings. At that time, her periods were beginning to be a little erratic but she now has a regular withdrawal bleed on HRT. She has been using condoms for contraception but her partner is experiencing some difficulty with them. She is terrified about the prospect of an unplanned pregnancy and asks her general practitioner about the possibility of being sterilized.

Her doctor sensibly advises her against a sterilization procedure as her natural fertility is very low and therefore an operative sterilization procedure is not warranted. Other methods to consider in conjunction with HRT would be an intrauterine device, the progestogen-only pill or a diaphragm.

Alison could continue with contraception until the age of 55 years when complete loss of fertility can be assumed. Alternatively, she could discontinue HRT for a period of 6–8 weeks and thereafter have an FSH level measured. If she does not menstruate spontaneously and has an FSH level greater than 30 IU/l then she should continue with contraception for one further year.

References

Barrington J, Bowen-Simpkins P (1997) The levonorgestrel intrauterine system in the management of menorrhagia. *Br J Obstet Gynaec* **104**: 614–16.

Carnall D (1995) Controvery rages over new contraceptive data. *Br Med J* **311**: 1117–18.

Collaborative Group on Hormonal Factors in Breast Cancer (1996) Breast cancer and hormonal contraceptives. *Lancet* **347**: 1713–27.

Coulter A, Kelland J, Long A et al. (1995) The management of menorrhagia. *Effective Health Care Bulletin.* Department of Health: London. (9): 2.

Cundy T, Evans M, Roberts H et al. (1991) Bone density in women receiving depot medroxyprogesterone acetate for contraception. *Br Med J* **30**: 13–16.

Gentile GP, Kaufman SC, Helbig DW (1998) Is there any evidence for a post-tubal sterilisation syndrome? *Fertil Steril* **69**: 179–86.

IPPF (1998) Statement on steroidal oral contraception. *IPPF Bull* **32**(6): 1–6.

Raudaskoski TH, Lahti EI, Kauppila AJ, Apaji-Sarkkinen MA, Laatikainen TJ (1995) Transdermal estrogen with a levonorgestrel-releasing intrauterine device for climacteric complaints: clinical and endometrial responses. *Am J Obstet Gynecol* **172**(1): 114–19.

Skegg D (1999) Oral contraception and health 1999 (editorial). *Br Med J* **318**: 69–70.

Tacchi D (1991) Long term use of copper intra-uterine devices. *Lancet* **336**: 182.

[WHO] World Health Organization Collaborative Study of Cardiovascular Disease and Steroid Hormone Contraception (1998) Cardiovascular disease and use of oral and injectable progestogen-only contraceptives and combined injectable contraceptives. Results of an international, multicenter, case-control study. *Contraception* **57**: 315–24.

Teenagers

Linda Egdell

Other chapters in this book cover contraception for people with a range of clinical conditions or specific problems. Teenagers are classified by age rather than by disease, and are among the healthiest of all potential contraceptive users.

Teenagers are among the healthiest of all contraceptive users

Society views teenagers as a 'problem', not least because of anxieties about the risk-taking behaviour of some young people. The widespread despondency about teenagers and their problems, including their media-sensationalized pregnancy rates, sometimes appear to deny the virtues and achievements of the vast majority of young men and women. Today's teenagers display confidence, enthusiasm, honesty, humour and often very caring personalities, making them a pleasure to work with.

What is a teenager?

Teenagers do not form a homogeneous group. Individual teenagers differ in their knowledge, values and experiences.

Age differences

The early teenage years are characterized by the physical and emotional changes of puberty. Worries about body changes, mood swings, self-absorption and rebellion are common. There is a need to conform with one's peers, and friendships—particularly with the same sex—are important. Very young teenagers may not be mature enough to take sensible decisions and can be vulnerable.

During the middle teens, with increasing emotional and intellectual maturity young people develop a set of personal values. Physical appearance becomes important. They embark upon relationships, albeit often of short duration but accompanied by strong feelings of attraction. Experimentation is common and the young person becomes physically and socially adventurous.

By the late teenage years young people regard themselves as adults, are becoming emotionally and financially independent, and may already have left home. They will tend to enter into longer-term relationships including cohabitation or marriage, and pregnancies may be planned and welcomed (Blackie et al. 1998).

Gender differences

In most societies today stereotypes of masculinity and femininity affect boys and girls in different ways. Young men have learned that maleness is equated with competitiveness and aggression whereas young women are expected to be passive and subordinate. Girls are, however, allowed to show feelings, to be more caring and to value romance in relationships (Aggleton et al. 1998).

Other factors

In addition to the obvious effects of age and gender, the unique experiences, knowledge, values and patterns of behaviour of each individual young person will have been influenced by a variety of factors. These will include socioeconomic and cultural background, religious constraints, academic achievement, and even factors such as residence in a rural as opposed to an urban setting (Smith 1993).

Teenage sexual activity

By the age of 20 years the majority of people in the Western world will already have had sexual intercourse. A survey of sexual attitudes and lifestyles of 18 876 British residents aged 16–59 years (Wellings et al. 1994) found that over the preceding four decades the median age at first intercourse fell by 4 years for women and 3 years for men to 17 years for both sexes. In this study 18.7% of the teenage women and 27.6% of the teenage men sampled stated that they had had sexual intercourse before the age of 16 years. These figures contrast with the results from the cohort aged 55–59 years where only 1% of women and 5.8% of men recalled having had their first sexual intercourse before the age of 16 years. Earlier studies (e.g. Farrell 1978) confirm this significant change over time.

Some recent reports paint a more alarming picture. A study by Burack (1999) of 1500 school pupils in London reported that 20% of 13-year-olds alleged that they had already experienced either full or oral sexual intercourse.

Even without considering the moral or legal implications of these trends, and the danger that young people who experiment at a very early age may come to regret their actions in later life, the risks in terms of pregnancies and sexually transmitted infections are of concern. Rates of sexually transmitted infections are highest among young people. Teenagers who embark on a sexual relationship before the age of 16 years are much less likely to use contraception (Mellanby et al. 1993, Lo et al. 1994).

Teenage conception rates

Figure 1 shows that the rate of conception (live and still births and terminations) to teenage girls in the UK has actually fallen substantially from the levels seen in the early 1970s. This is presumably because of the availability of the oral contraceptive pill and easier access by young unmarried women to contraceptive services that were absorbed into the National Health Service in 1974. There was a small increase in the 1980s, followed by a drop between 1990 and 1995 from 69 to 59 per 1000 girls aged 15–19 years. Levels then began to rise again, reflecting a similar trend across older age groups and coinciding with the October 1995 pill alert about an association between venous thromboembolism and certain progestogens. The conception rate in 1996 was 63 per 1000 girls aged 15–19 years.

More than a third of all pregnancies in teenage girls in the UK are terminated and the abortion rate is currently rising (Office for National Statistics).

For girls under 16 years old, conception rates remained at a fairly constant level for 30 years up to 1996, in which year 9.4 out of every 1000 girls aged 13–15 years became pregnant. Half of the pregnancies in this age group are terminated.

Abortion can cause medical and emotional effects. Concerns about young women who continue their pregnancies centre around the increased risks to maternal and fetal health and the social disadvantages of being a teenage mother. Pregnant teenagers are more likely to

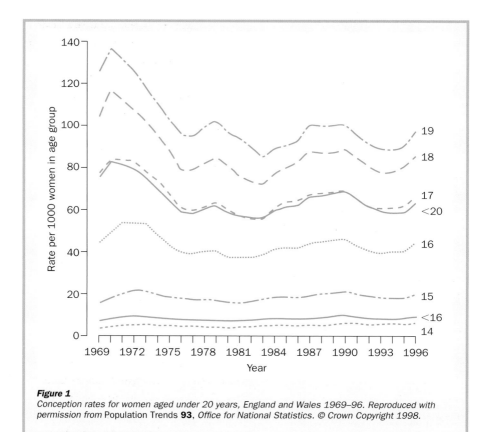

Figure 1
Conception rates for women aged under 20 years, England and Wales 1969–96. Reproduced with permission from Population Trends **93**, Office for National Statistics. © Crown Copyright 1998.

suffer anaemia and pre-eclampsia, partly because they can be poor attenders for antenatal care and also because of the socially disadvantaged backgrounds that predisposed to the early pregnancy in the first place. The babies themselves are at risk through higher rates of perinatal mortality, lower birthweights and a higher incidence of certain congenital abnormalities. Teenage mothers can face isolation, economic and other social disadvantages, almost certain disruption to their education and a continuing cycle of deprivation. This will in turn affect their babies and the young fathers too if they choose to remain within the family unit (Irvine et al. 1997, Botting et al. 1998).

Factors affecting teenage pregnancy rates

The reasons why some teenage girls are more likely to become pregnant than others are complex and interlinked.

Geographical differences

Teenage pregnancy rates are not spread evenly across the UK. Government advice in the Green Paper *Our Healthier Nation* (1998) has now changed the previous blanket target of halving of the rates in girls under 16 years old by the year 2000 to advising instead that agencies should address the issue if there is a particular problem locally.

More striking than locally different rates within the UK are the international variations.

Rates of teenage pregnancy in the UK are three times as high as those in the Netherlands

Teenage pregnancy rates in the UK are the highest in Western Europe. Comparing six Western industrialized nations, Jones et al. (1986) found that in the Netherlands rates of only one-third of those in the UK had been achieved, whereas the rates in the USA were double. Cultural differences may be a factor. However, common threads in countries where teenage pregnancies have been successfully reduced include an open, tolerant and pragmatic attitude to sexuality, effective programmes of sex education, and access to confidential and appropriate contraceptive services (Peckham 1993, Ketting 1993, Nyman 1993).

Socioeconomic disadvantage and family background

Garlick et al. (1993) compared teenage pregnancy rates in different health authority areas in one health region and found significantly higher rates where the underprivileged area scores—a marker for poverty—were high. The need to target contraceptive services at those areas of greatest deprivation was highlighted. Other studies have shown that teenage girls from broken homes, those who have been in care or come from a large family, girls who truant from school and those who were themselves the daughters of teenage mothers are more likely to become pregnant.

Academic achievement

Young women who have higher educational attainments, who stay on at school and who have parents who are supportive and interested in their education are less likely to become pregnant (Effective Health Care 1997).

Levels of knowledge

Arguments against provision of school-based sex education include the charge that giving young people information will make them more likely to experiment. This was refuted in the study by Wellings et al. (1994) which showed that respondents to a questionnaire for whom school had been the main source of their knowledge were less likely to have had sexual intercourse before the age of 16 years and were more likely to have used contraception.

Studies from the USA of different models of sex education indicate that the most effective programmes may be those that are linked to vocational guidance, those that convey factual information on local services and with links to local or school-based clinics, approaches using individual counselling or peer-led groups, and those that build up confidence and assertiveness skills. By comparison, programmes that concentrated solely on teaching abstinence from sexual activity were less likely to be successful (Effective Health Care 1997).

Availability of contraceptive services

Access to appropriate contraceptive services for sexually active teenagers is certainly important. However, increasing the provision of contraceptive services alone does not necessarily lower conception or abortion rates. Wilson et al. (1992) compared teenage pregnancy rates, attendance at local family planning clinics and standardized mortality ratios (SMRs) in the English health regions. It was concluded that effective programmes to tackle social disadvantage would confer greater benefit than simply providing more clinics.

Contraceptive services for young people

Measures to address social inequalities, and provision of effective programmes of sex education, are the responsibility of governments.

Health authorities and individual practitioners are responsible for providing effective services that teenagers will want to use. Much work has been done in defining what constitutes a clinically effective service for young people.

In their 1992 guidelines to the UK health regions for reviewing family planning services, the NHS Executive referred to the Department of Health circular HC(86)1 which advocated 'separate, less formal arrangements for young people'. This can be achieved in various settings appropriate to local needs; different models of service may have equal validity and presenting choice to young people can only maximize uptake. Reviewing existing provision, assessing local need and involving a wide range of relevant agencies and groups are all valuable when planning services.

A study of two general practices in Devon (Pereira Gray and Seamark 1995) found that more than half of the female teenage population of the practices had consulted the general practitioner for contraceptive advice. There are several advantages, not only that of proximity to the surgery, for young people in using their general practitioner. The surgery is open for most of the week, the primary health-care team will be aware of the young person's background and medical history, and since people consult general practitioners for a wide range of purposes the teenager's reason for attending will not be obvious to others in the waiting room. However, lessons can be learned from some of the research into factors affecting young people's willingness to approach traditional services.

In a study of three young people's projects (Allen 1991), half of the teenagers aged 16–19 years who were interviewed said they feared

that a visit to the general practitioner for contraception would not remain confidential. Three-quarters of interviewees under 16 years old voiced the same concerns. Concerns about confidentiality and a possible unfriendly reception were reasons cited in another study (Donovan et al. 1997) for some young teenagers' reluctance to consult their general practitioner. Again, a paper on teenage contraceptive services and the need for family planning clinics (Allaby 1995) showed that conception rates were lowest in those Oxford health districts where a higher proportion of all users of contraceptive services had attended community family planning clinics. This study concluded that, particularly for those under 16 years old, teenage contraceptive services may be more effective in areas where clinics play a major part in the service delivery.

Confidentiality of contraceptive services is the most important consideration for most young people

Protocols for delivering contraceptive services to young people, whatever the model of provision, should take heed of the views of young people.

The services young people want

Studies such as those of Allen (1991), Wardle and Wright (1993) and others have shown that several factors affect teenagers' use of contraceptive services. Many young people are attracted to the idea of their own clinic, but a convenient location is important. They like local but discreet clinics which are easy to find but not too conspicuous (*Figure 2*). Large clinical health settings are less liked, as are crowded waiting areas where young people could be observed by family members or neighbours. They prefer to attend during the evening or at weekends. They appreciate drop-in services or appointments that are immediate and easy to arrange. Magazines and drinks are welcomed and decor should be attractive. A young person often attends with several friends for support and may feel much more confident if invited to bring them into the consulting room.

Views about the professionals approved of by young people are clear. They particularly want to see staff who, although expert and professional, are nonetheless friendly and easy to talk to. Teenagers fear disapproval, interrogation and rejection and do not like being told what to do. It is very important to treat young people with respect and dignity; not to lecture or to reject. Some young women prefer to see a female practitioner for embarrassing examinations but the sex of the doctor or nurse is less important than attitude (Brook Advisory Centres 1998).

A relaxed, 'trendy', informal atmosphere is thought by professionals to be important. However, one young girl said, 'We don't really mind whether you wear white coats or not. We don't even care if you are very old. What we don't like is being asked too many questions, being told off and being asked how old we are' (personal communication).

Professionals are equally sure that services must be widely publicized and advise spending a great deal of money on advertising. However, most attenders at young people's clinics do not seem to have seen the posters but say instead that the service was recommended to them by friends. This may be why a new service can take time to become popular.

In a survey of clinic attenders in Eastbourne and Ipswich (Jones 1996) the majority were in favour of combining family planning and genitourinary medicine services into a 'one-stop shop' sexual health service. Young people were the most enthusiastic supporters of this.

Young men are not good users of contraceptive services even when these are specifically for young people. They may well have had less comprehensive sex education,

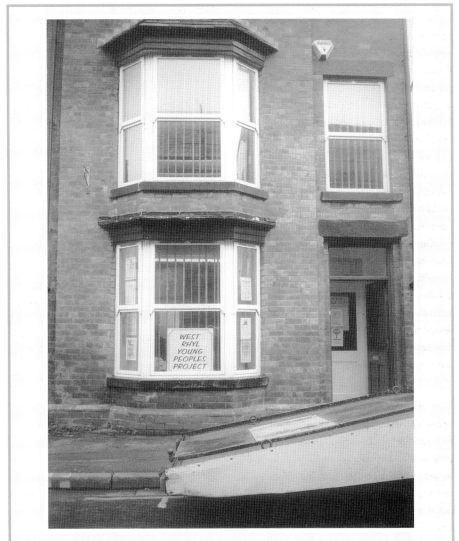

Figure 2
Young people like local but discreet clinics which are easy to find but not too conspicuous (West Rhyl Young People's Project).

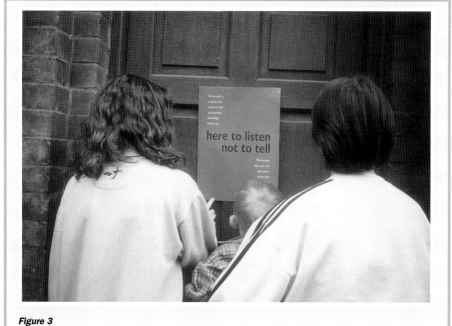

Figure 3
Reassurance about the confidential nature of the service is important (poster for the Brook Advisory Centres).

may feel that contraception is the girl's responsibility, do not see the need to protect themselves, and prefer the anonymity of slot machines for condoms. Some innovative schemes whereby young men can obtain condoms and advice from youth workers and young people's projects can be successful.

The single most important consideration for young people is a firm stated reassurance about the confidential nature of the service (*Figure 3*).

Confidentiality and young people

Article 16 of the 1991 United Nations Convention on the Rights of the Child, which defined minimum standards for legislation, policies and practice affecting children up to the age of 18 years, guarantees the child's right to privacy. Teenagers, like older adults, are entitled to have their sexual lives kept private, and even where teenagers have a good relationship with their parents they usually do not wish to disclose to them intimate details of their current relationships.

Guidance issued jointly by the British Medical Association and its General Medical Services Committee, the Health Education Authority, Brook Advisory Centres, the Family Planning Association and the Royal College of General Practitioners (*Confidentiality and People Under 16*) states that 'the duty of confidentiality owed to a person under 16 is as great as that owed to any other person'. In defining good medical practice, the guidance highlights the task of educating young people about the confidentiality they can expect from their doctor, and advises: 'establishing a trusting relationship between the patient and the doctor at this stage will do more to promote health than if doctors refuse to see young patients without involving parents'.

However, no patient of any age has an absolute right to confidentiality. There may be a need to protect vulnerable people from harm, for example in situations of abuse, and child protection implications must always be considered. If, in rare circumstances, confidentiality is to be breached the doctor must first seek permission from the patient

and then be prepared to justify the decision before the General Medical Council.

The law and contraceptive advice to children under 16 years old

The document quoted from above also states: 'any *competent* young person, regardless of age, can independently seek medical advice and give valid consent to treatment'.

Following the 1985 House of Lords ruling in the Gillick case, the Department of Health restated the factors that doctors and other professionals need to consider before providing contraceptive advice and treatment to young people under 16 (circular HC(86)1). The importance of not undermining parental responsibility and family stability, the need for separate less formal arrangements, and the importance of trained experienced staff were all cited. In acknowledging that there will be cases where it is not possible to persuade the young person to involve the parents, this circular permits doctors and other professionals to give advice and treatment to competent patients under 16 years old without parental knowledge or consent. However, the practitioner may only do this provided that the five conditions, as ruled by the Law Lords in their judgement in 1985, are fulfilled (see box).

When approached, clinicians must be prepared to assume responsibility and to

DEPARTMENT OF HEALTH GUIDANCE IN 1986 ABOUT THE PROVISION OF CONTRACEPTIVE ADVICE AND TREATMENT TO YOUNG PEOPLE UNDER 16 YEARS OLD

A doctor or other professional would be justified in giving contraceptive advice and treatment to a young person under 16 without parental knowledge and consent provided he was satisfied:

1. *that the young person could understand his advice and had sufficient maturity to understand what was involved in terms of the moral social and emotional implications*
2. *that he could neither persuade the young person to inform the parents, nor to allow him to inform them, that contraceptive advice was being sought*
3. *that the young person would be very likely to begin, or to continue, having sexual intercourse with or without contraceptive treatment*
4. *that without contraceptive advice or treatment, the young person's physical or mental health, or both, would be likely to suffer*
5. *that the young person's best interests required him to give contraceptive advice, treatment or both without parental consent*

consider offering protection. It is often useful to discuss with the youngster the relationship that exists with her or his parents, and to explore whether the parents might already be expressing concern. Attending for contraception is a responsible action and the teenager deserves praise. Teenagers often say that they intend to tell their mothers themselves at the right time.

Contraceptive care for teenagers

As will be apparent from the previous sections in this chapter there is a large amount of published evidence about teenage sexual activity, pregnancy rates and the reasons for them, and much data to support the need for effective services. There is, however, less documented material about contraceptive care that is appropriate for young people once they are inside the consulting room, and the types of contraception that might be suitable for them.

Patterns of use of services

The first approach by a teenager to a doctor or clinic is all too often only made in a crisis. A study of 205 young people making their first visit to two separate young people's clinics in North Wales showed that 53 (26%) attended for emergency contraception, a further 38 (19%) feared they could be pregnant and were requesting a test, and 4 (2%) already knew that they were pregnant and were seeking abortion (Collins A, Egdell L, 1998, unpublished observation). Only 12 (6%) were not already sexually active at the time of their first visit. Young people could be helped by a discussion of the benefits in allowing relationships to develop slowly, in delaying sex until they are sure and in learning the skills to negotiate if and when to have sex and to obtain contraception beforehand. One pregnant 15-year-old girl, when asked if she had mentioned using a condom to her boyfriend of three weeks, said 'I couldn't possibly talk to him about things like that'.

The attitude of the clinician towards a young girl who presents because she has failed to use contraception is important. She is usually apprehensive and expects to be lectured. Perhaps instead she should be praised for her courage and sense in attending. Once the immediate crisis is dealt with, staff can then take the opportunity presented to help her take better care of herself in the future.

The experience in many clinics is that young people tend to use services spasmodically and unpredictably. They will present during the emergency but may well not be seen again until another panic occurs. Any contraception provided is often abandoned as the teenager moves in and out of brief relationships. Of the 205 clients followed up in the North Wales clinics, 120 (59%) had not returned by 6 months after the end of the 12-month recruiting period. The other 85 (41%) had reattended at least once and 17 (8%) made five or more visits. Services should recognize these patterns and be flexible and innovative. At one of the clinics in North Wales, held in a multi-agency, multi-purpose young people's centre, advice, free condoms and pregnancy testing are available from youth workers throughout the week. More young people avail themselves of this service than attend the weekly clinic.

Contraceptive consultations for young people

As with all family planning consultations, establishing the reason for attendance and careful history-taking are important. Knowledge and previous experience of contraceptive methods should be elicited and a sexual history sensitively taken. A general medical and family history will exclude contraindications to certain contraceptives, but teenagers can be hazy about previous illnesses, medication or reasons for hospitalization, and may not know much about the health of the immediate family. A clinician who is not the patient's usual doctor should seek permission from the girl to obtain this information from her general practitioner before proceeding to treat.

Allowing adequate time for counselling will facilitate discussion about relationships, sexually transmitted infections and general health concerns. Wider health promotion about sensible eating and advice on smoking, drugs and alcohol are also appropriate.

Information about all methods of contraception, including benefits and risks, mode of use and reliability, will help the young person to make an informed choice. If the young woman has brought her partner he should be involved in the decisions (Hadley 1990).

Most reversible methods can be considered for young, fit women. A low-dose combined pill has non-contraceptive advantages particularly for irregular menstrual cycles, premenstrual symptoms and heavy painful periods. Running packets together to avoid menstruation during school examinations or while on holiday can be beneficial.

Nevertheless, young girls often fear the pill. They may be put off by concerns about weight gain, or worry that their mothers will find the pill packet. They may doubt whether they will remember to take it, or just feel that the relationship is not yet sufficiently secure

and intercourse too infrequent for the commitment of the pill.

The effectiveness of the combined pill depends upon good compliance. In practice, 'typical use' may lead to pregnancy rates of 3% to 20%—far greater than the rate from 'perfect use' (International Working Group 1993, Trussell et al. 1996). Teenage girls are particularly at risk of conceiving because of missed pills.

The effectiveness of the COC depends upon good compliance. Teenagers are particularly at risk of conceiving because of missed pills

If a teenage girl opts to take the pill the blood pressure should be measured. Any other routine examination or investigation is usually unnecessary and is best avoided. Cervical smears are not indicated in women under 20 years old, but the role of human papilloma virus in cervical cancer and the importance of condom use to prevent it should be discussed.

It is important to choose a brand of pill which is well packaged and easy to swallow. The girl may have to consider how to hide her pills at home without forgetting them. Some pill packets contain user-friendly instruction booklets. Phasic pills are more complicated than monophasic brands. Some teenagers like to take the pill used by their friends or sisters. The method should be carefully taught using a sample packet and backed up by leaflets. Recall of the instructions and compliance should be checked at early follow-up.

Progestogen-only pills which must be taken regularly are less suitable in this age group. On the other hand, non-oral hormonal contraceptives can be very successful because they are discreet and do not rely on the user's memory. The injectable method is gaining in popularity among young women but clinicians may need to establish a confidential means of communication if repeat appointments are missed. Progestogen implants can be ideal because of their long-term action. Although difficult to insert into a nulliparous uterus the progestogen-loaded intrauterine system could be considered, because it appears to carry a reduced risk of pelvic inflammatory disease.

Copper-bearing intrauterine devices may be suitable but only where the risk of sexually transmitted infections is very low. The frameless intrauterine implant may be better tolerated in the nulliparous uterus. Pre-insertion screening for infection including chlamydia should be considered.

A few young women in stable relationships may choose the diaphragm. Consistent use is necessary to achieve good efficacy. The nonoxynol 9 in the spermicidal cream used with the cap may be bactericidal and viricidal. If the girl does not live with her boyfriend she may have practical problems in storing and transporting her device.

Male and female condoms offer protection against infection and can be used in conjunction with another method. Most young people are fully aware of the protective effect of condoms and acknowledge that they should be used in all new relationships. Negotiating their use during sex is less easy. Young couples will abandon condoms after a while because they like to think they can now 'trust each other' and the girl may have commenced taking the pill. Counselling in this situation needs sensitivity because logically every couple—even older long-married ones—should also always use condoms! Why should the young be singled out? In practice it may be helpful to encourage continuing with condoms in case pills are forgotten, and also to allow the male to take some of the responsibility. Condom usage should be taught by someone prepared to discuss details of the sexual relationship.

Some teenagers are attracted by the technology of personal ovulation indicators. The need to follow the rules about when to abstain and the lower effectiveness of natural methods should be stressed.

Whichever method is chosen the teenager should also be given information about emergency contraception. Young people are more aware of the existence of the 'morning after' pill than some older people. They are often not sure about the correct time limits and may not know where to obtain it (Graham et al. 1996).

It is important that young people are informed about the availability of emergency contraception

The pregnant teenager

If pregnancy is suspected early diagnosis is important. All young people's services should offer on-the-spot pregnancy testing. For reasons of fear, denial or disbelief some teenagers may conceal their pregnancies and present late.

When a pregnancy is confirmed the girl needs support in deciding what to do. She may be reluctant to tell her parents, fearing their anger and disappointment or trying to protect her partner. An abortion may be requested solely so that the parents will never know. Girls under 16 years old who are competent can undergo an abortion without parental consent but must have practical and emotional support from someone at this time. Usually they find the courage to get this from their mothers or perhaps another family member.

If the teenager continues with her pregnancy she may need help with her finances, housing and education. Her social, emotional and health needs should be addressed. In some areas comprehensive services for pregnant teenagers have been established. There are units with crèches where education can be continued, often linked to teenage antenatal and postnatal clinics. Other young girls are happy to visit the midwife at their local surgery. With support to the teenager the arrival of her new baby can bring much happiness into the family.

Working with teenagers

Helping young people with their relationships, contraception and sexual health requires aptitude, interest and training. It is also fun and can be very rewarding. It is a privilege to follow teenagers through the turmoils and uncertainties of adolescence, to play a part in their learning process as they fall in love, develop caring relationships and avoid some of the pitfalls and finally to witness their successful transition to adulthood with plans to look after families of their own.

Case histories

Case 1

Emma, who is 15-years-old, attends a young people's clinic because she has not had a period for a few months. A pregnancy test is positive and examination confirms an 18 week pregnancy.

Emma has had sex only once, about four months ago with a transient boyfriend. The following afternoon she presented at the Accident and Emergency Department of her local hospital, asking for emergency contraception. It was very busy there but she was eventually seen by a doctor. She says he seemed cross with her and told her off. She thinks he said that the emergency pill could be dangerous because it was very strong, and he certainly told her that she would not be seen again without her mother. However, he gave her the emergency pills anyway. When Emma got home she swallowed two of the pills and later felt very sick and unwell. She did not take the second dose.

'He got it wrong. His pills made me ill and didn't work,' she says.

When her period did not arrive a friend assured her that the emergency pill could delay things. More recently, another friend thought she could have a 'blockage'. Emma confided in the school nurse who sent her to the clinic.

Emma needs her confidence in the medical profession restored but this is a long-term project. She is referred for consideration of mid-trimester termination and associated counselling and given an appointment to return to the clinic in the future.

Case 2

Sarah, aged 17 years, attends the family planning clinic with her mother, who has herself attended for many years. Sarah and her mother have a good relationship and sex has always been discussed openly in the family. Sarah is in sixth form college and hopes to study languages at university. Her parents are proud of her and very supportive.

When Sarah and her boyfriend Craig, who have been together for over a year, decided they would start having sex they agreed that Sarah should first go on the pill. So Sarah spoke to her mother who volunteered to accompany her daughter to the clinic. 'I knew I'd be sitting here with her one day,' her mother says. Sarah is happy to use condoms as well as the pill. She is encouraged to bring Craig with her to her next appointment, rather than her mother.

Case 3

Rachel is only just 14 years old and pregnant. She comes from a large family. Two younger siblings have special needs. Rachel herself has been excluded from school because of behavioural problems. Her mother, who was only 16 years old herself when she gave birth to Rachel's older sister, had to get married. She wants Rachel to have an abortion. The house is too small for them all as it is and Rachel's mother does not want to give up her factory job to look after a grandchild. Rachel's father, who is unemployed, is refusing to discuss the pregnancy. He has 'washed his hands of her'.

Rachel does not know who the father is. She thinks it could be one of four different men. She and her friend are much more interested in when the baby is likely to be born.

Her mother brings her to the surgery to talk about having an abortion, but Rachel thinks a baby would be nice. She would like to look after it and play with it. She says that all her friends have already offered to baby-sit. She thinks that her older sister should leave home to make more room. She is adamant that she is going to go through with the pregnancy.

Rachel's plans need to be respected, however naïve they may appear. She is referred for antenatal care but also given a contact number should she wish to change her mind and request a termination. The family is already well known to Social Services.

References

Aggleton P, Oliver C, Rivers K (1998) *The Implications of Research into Young People, Sex, Sexuality and Relationships.* London: Health Education Authority, University of London.

Allaby A (1995) Contraceptive services for teenagers: do we need family planning clinics? *Br Med J* 310: 1641–3.

Allen I (1991) *Family Planning and Pregnancy Counselling Projects for Young People.* London: Policy Studies Institute.

Blackie C, Greg R, Freeth D (1998) Promoting health in young people. *Nursing Standard* 12(36): 39–46.

Botting B, Rosato M, Wood R (1998) Teenage mothers and the health of their children. *Population Trends* 93, pp 19–28. London: Office for National Statistics.

Brook Advisory Centres (1998) *Someone With a Smile Would Be Your Best Bet.* London: Brook Advisory Publications.

Burack R (1999) Teenage sexual behaviour: attitudes towards and declared sexual activity. *Br J Fam Plan* 24: 145–8.

Donovan C, Mellanby A, Jacobsen L, Taylor B, Tripp J (1997) Teenagers' views on the general practice consultation and provision of contraception. The Adolescent Working Group. *Br J Gen Pract* 47(424): 715–18.

Effective Health Care (1997) *Preventing and Reducing the Adverse Effects of Unintended Teenage Pregnancies.* University of York: NHS Centres for Reviews and Dissemination.

Farrell C (1978) *My Mother Said . . .* London: Routledge & Kegan Paul.

Garlick R, Ineichen B, Hudson F (1993) The UPA score and teenage pregnancy. *Publ Health* 107: 135–9.

Graham A, Green L, Glasier A (1996) Teenagers' knowledge of emergency contraception: questionnaire survey in south east Scotland. *Br Med J* 312: 1567–9.

Hadley A (1990) Contraception for the young. *Community Outlook* March.

International Working Group (1993) A consensus statement: enhancing patient compliance and oral contraceptive efficacy. *Br J Fam Plan* 18: 126–9.

Irvine H, Bradley T, Cupples M, Boohan M (1997) The implications of teenage pregnancy and motherhood for primary health care: unresolved issues. *Br J Gen Pract* 47: 323–6.

Jones E, Forrest J, Goldman N (1986) *Teenage Pregnancy in Industrialized Countries.* New York: Yale University Press.

Jones M (1996) Clients expressing preference for one-stop sexual health shop. *Nursing Times* 92: 32–3.

Ketting E (1993) The Dutch experience of teenage pregnancy—lessons for Wales. *Teenage Pregnancy: Proceedings of a One-day International Seminar in West Glamorgan*, pp 26–29. Swansea: Department of Public Health Medicine, West Glamorgan Health Authority.

Lo S, Kaul S, Kaul R, Cooling S, Calvert J (1994) Teenage pregnancy—contraceptive use and non-use. *Br J Fam Plan* 20: 79–83.

Mellanby A, Phelps F, Tripp J (1993) Teenagers, sex and risk taking. *Br Med J* 307: 25.

Nyman V (1993) Going Dutch—a pipe dream? *Br J Fam Plan* 19: 200–3.

Peckham S (1993) Preventing unintended teenage pregnancies. *Publ Health* 107: 125–33.

Pereira Gray D, Seamark C (1995) Do teenagers consult general practitioners for contraceptive advice? *Br J Fam Plan* 21: 50–1.

Smith T (1993) Influence of socio-economic factors on attaining targets for reducing teenage pregnancies. *Br Med J* 306: 1232–5.

Trussell J, Steiner M, Dominik R, Hertz-Picciott I (1996) Measuring contraceptive effectiveness: a conceptual framework. *Obstet Gynaecol* 88(Suppl): 245–305.

Wardle S, Wright P (1993) Family planning services—the needs of young people. A report from Mid Staffordshire. *Br J Fam Plan* 19: 158–60.

Wellings K, Wadsworth J, Johnson AM, Field J (1994) *Sexual Attitudes and Lifestyles.* Oxford: Blackwell Scientific.

Wilson S, Brown T, Richards R (1992) Teenage conception and contraception in the English regions. *J Publ Health Med* 14: 17–25.

Women with polycystic ovaries

Stephen Killick and Michael O'Connell

8

Polycystic ovary syndrome (PCOS) is a complex but common endocrine condition in which a characteristic polycystic appearance of the ovaries is associated with clinical features such as oligomenorrhoea, hyperandrogenism, subfertility and obesity.

Women with PCOS not only suffer a variety of distressing symptoms but also have specific long-term health risks. By sheer good fortune the non-contraceptive effects of certain forms of hormonal contraception can be beneficial for both the immediate symptoms and the long-term health of women with PCOS. The recognition of women who have polycystic ovaries and advice given to them about their contraceptive choices are an important part of the work of family planning doctors.

Polycystic ovary syndrome

PCOS is extremely variable in its clinical features and biochemical characteristics. Generally speaking there is a raised serum concentration of luteinizing hormone (LH) which stimulates excessive androgen production from the ovarian stroma (*Figure 1*), and most of the clinical and biochemical features can be explained in terms of an abundance of androgenic hormones. It is not always possible, however, to demonstrate abnormally high serum androgen concentrations or even a

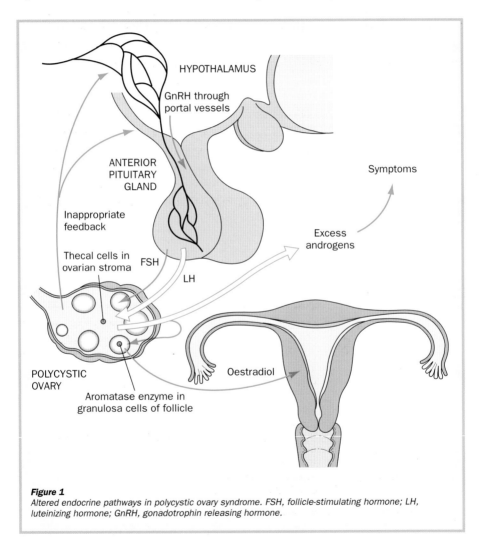

Figure 1
Altered endocrine pathways in polycystic ovary syndrome. FSH, follicle-stimulating hormone; LH, luteinizing hormone; GnRH, gonadotrophin releasing hormone.

raised LH level. Not surprisingly, some authorities do not consider these cases to be true PCOS. No single structural or biochemical abnormality is pathognomonic and attempts to produce a working definition for clinical or research purposes have used a combination of ovarian morphology, endocrine values and clinical features.

Symptoms usually develop gradually and can arise at any age after the menarche—most commonly in the late teens and early twenties. Women present with a continuously variable spectrum of symptoms (*Table 1*), from a mild menstrual irregularity to the fat, hairy,

amenorrhoeic, infertile women as originally described over sixty years ago (Stein and Leventhal 1935). It is interesting to note, however, that the symptoms of an individual woman rarely change except to become gradually more severe as the years go by. Similarly, in the situation where the syndrome seems to run in a family, the individual family members suffer similar symptoms. The syndrome appears to have a genetic origin although the details are unknown. It is possible, of course, that the syndrome represents several different genetic conditions. In one form the hyperandrogenism seems to be inherited from

Table 1
Symptoms, signs and long-term health risks of polycystic ovary syndrome.

Symptoms	Signs	Long-term health risks
Oligomenorrhoea	Polycystic ovaries	Risks of obesity
Amenorrhoea	Raised serum LH	Type II diabetes mellitus
Subfertility	LH : FSH ratio > 3 : 1	Endometrial carcinoma
Obesity	Anovulation	Coronary artery disease
Hirsutism	Increased waist to hip ratio	Hypertension
Acne	Hyperandrogenaemia	Possibly breast carcinoma
Male-pattern alopecia	Hyperinsulinaemia	
Pelvic pain	Hyperlipidaemia	
Recurrent miscarriage	Hyperprolactinaemia	
	Low SHBG	

LH, luteinizing hormone; FSH, follicle-stimulating hormone; SHBG, sex hormone binding globulin.

the father who phenotypically has premature baldness.

Ovarian morphological features of PCOS

Stein and Leventhal (1935) described enlarged ovaries with thick 'sclerocystic' capsules. However, ovarian biopsy is obviously undesirable as a diagnostic test and laparoscopic appearances are extremely subjective. Ultrasound appearances have been shown to correlate well with the histopathological studies (Saxton et al. 1990) and therefore ultrasound has replaced the laparoscope as the main diagnostic tool in the evaluation of PCOS.

Polycystic ovaries are usually said to be those that are enlarged and contain more than ten cysts, 2–8 mm in diameter, situated peripherally around an echo-dense, thickened central stroma (Adams et al. 1985) (*Figure 2*). This definition, however, has not remained static because the resolving power of ovarian imaging techniques has increased. Swanson, using transabdominal ultrasound, originally described a characteristic appearance without a quantified number of cysts (Swanson et al. 1981). More recently vaginal ultrasonography has suggested fifteen peripheral cysts to be a more appropriate definition, and the use of three-dimensional ultrasound and magnetic resonance imaging (Kimura et al. 1996) will overdiagnose the

condition because of the more accurate ovarian images unless the definition is similarly modified (*Figure 3*). Unfortunately, this means that many ultrasound departments do not have a standard morphological definition for what is and what is not a polycystic ovary.

Many ultrasound departments do not have a standard morphological definition for what is and what is not a polycystic ovary

All women with PCOS have ovaries that appear polycystic. However, even allowing for the variations caused by different ovarian imaging techniques, it is apparent that many women with ovaries that are structurally polycystic are completely asymptomatic and do not have a clinical problem. Using the Adams definition referred to above, the prevalence of polycystic ovaries (PCO) in premenopausal asymptomatic women is as high as 23% (Polson et al. 1988). It seems unlikely that these women have the same long-term health risks as those with PCOS and it is therefore important to differentiate between PCO and PCOS.

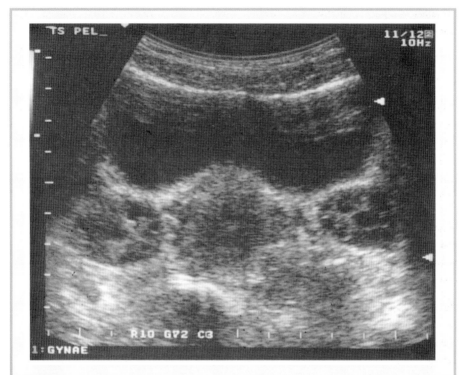

Figure 2
Transabdominal ultrasound view of a polycystic ovary. Taken from a woman with infertility about to undergo ovulation induction. Note the peripheral cystic structures and the central stroma.

It is important to distinguish between PCO and PCOS

One further diagnostic trap for those wishing to diagnose PCOS using ultrasound is the multicystic ovary (*Figure 4*). Multicystic ovaries also contain multiple cysts 4–10 mm in diameter but in contrast to polycystic ovaries the stromal volume is not increased (Polson et al. 1988). This type of ovary is seen in adolescent girls and in women recovering from weight-related amenorrhoea. It represents an ovarian response to reduced or immature pituitary stimulation.

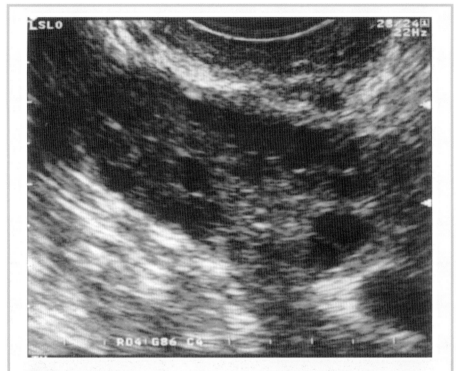

Figure 3
Nuclear magnetic resonance (NMR) view of a polycystic ovary. Taken from an obese woman with subfertility and oligomenorrhoea. Note the cysts are apparently more abundant than in Figure 2 because of the increased resolution of NMR compared to ultrasound. Image courtesy of Professor Lindsay Turnbull, NMR Centre, University of Hull.

Hormonal features of PCOS

Polycystic ovary syndrome is associated with increased serum concentrations of LH, oestradiol, prolactin and androgen, but, in contrast to the structural changes in the ovary, some or all of these features may not be present. This often leads to confusion with the diagnosis.

Definitions have included such features as a ratio of luteinizing hormone to follicle-stimulating hormone (LH : FSH) greater than 3 : 1, or an exaggerated LH response to

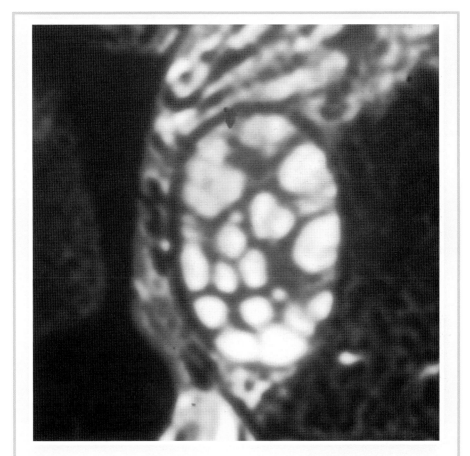

Figure 4
An NMR view of multicystic ovaries. Taken from a woman with weight-related amenorrhoea. Note the relative lack of stromal tissue compared with Figure 3. Image courtesy of Professor Lindsay Turnbull, NMR Centre, University of Hull.

gonadotrophin releasing hormone (GnRH). More recently the GnRH agonist test has been used to define PCOS (Ehrmann et al. 1995).

In 80% of patients with the clinical phenotype of PCOS the response of 17α-OH-progesterone and androstenedione were both excessive. The biological hyperandrogenism of PCOS cannot be used to define the syndrome because in most cases the serum levels of androstenedione and testosterone are moderately and inconsistently elevated in a non-specific manner. Suppression of serum levels of sex hormone binding globulin (SHBG) occurs in 40–50% of cases of PCOS and so leads to an increase in free serum testosterone.

A useful definition of PCOS

The 1990 National Institutes of Health–National Institute of Child Health and Development (NIH–NICHD) consensus conference achieved an empirical definition suggesting that clinical symptoms (hyperandrogenism and/or anovulation) should serve as the selecting criteria and hormone results should exclude 'anything that is not PCOS'. The advantages are that it is simple, economic and safe. This definition does not include ultrasound criteria and so excludes controversial asymptomatic cases.

Clinical features—and how contraceptive hormones may help

Hyperandrogenism

The hyperandrogenic component of the syndrome consists of increased male hair-growth pattern, acne and seborrhoea; in essence, mild androgenic stimulation of the pilosebaceous unit. The symptom of male-pattern alopecia is less common and usually occurs in more severe cases.

Increased hair growth on the upper lip, arms, abdomen and legs is socially unacceptable in many parts of the English-speaking world and women often complain bitterly of hirsutism, even in cases so mild that the physician is unable to confirm the diagnosis objectively. Race and naturally dark hair colouring may contribute to the problem although 70% of cases of hirsutism are thought to be the result of PCOS (Balen et al. 1995).

All forms of hormonal contraception, to a greater or lesser extent, suppress gonadotrophin release from the pituitary gland. Luteinizing hormone is the main stimulator of androgen production by the theca cells so any effective hormonal contraceptive should go some way to alleviate the hyperandrogenism of PCOS. The effect is not usually great enough for most symptomatic women, however, and one problem is that many contraceptive progestogens are androgenic in their own right.

Combined oral contraceptives have been used extensively and successfully for women with PCOS (Azziz and Gay 1989, McKenna 1991, Delahunt 1993). Their effectiveness in suppressing the androgenic features is thought to be due to a combination of factors:

1. The secretion of LH by the pituitary is suppressed and hence there is less androgen production by the theca cells of the ovary.

2. Adrenal androgen production and secretion are suppressed by ethinyloestradiol.

3. Ethinyloestradiol increases serum SHBG, which leads to a decrease in free biologically active plasma testosterone.

The pharmaceutical industry has invested huge resources since the 1970s in producing progestogens of lower androgenicity, such as gestodene, desogestrel and norgestimate. Cyproterone, nomegestrol and dienogest are progestogens with antiandrogenic properties and are specifically marketed for their effects on acne and hirsutism.

Porcile and Gallardo (1991) reported a statistically significant improvement in hirsutism (objectively recorded by a decrease in Ferriman–Gallway–Lorenzo hair score) when hirsute patients were treated with either Marvelon (containing desogestrel) or Diane-35 (containing cyproterone). It is important to note that this study was conducted over a 2-year period and patients should be made fully aware of the time interval of 3–6 months prior to the onset of any symptomatic relief from hirsutism.

The newer progestogens are also more effective in resolving or improving acne. A randomized study comparing combined pills containing either desogestrel or levonorgestrel demonstrated a statistically significant improvement in the desogestrel group (Palatsi et al. 1984). Gestodene-containing pills are at least as good as desogestrel-containing pills for this purpose (Mango et al. 1996) and a multicentre study of women treated with norgestimate also showed a decrease in acne (Runnebaum 1992). However, as might be expected, pills containing one of the antiandrogenic progestogens such as cyproterone (Falsetti and Galbignani 1990) are the most useful for women with androgenic symptoms. Although these data refer to combined oral preparations, non-oral preparations such as monthly injections, patches or vaginal rings could be expected to be just as useful.

Oligomenorrhoea

It is reported that 87% of women with oligomenorrhoea have PCOS (Gonzales et al. 1988) and PCOS is also one of the most frequent causes of secondary amenorrhoea (Franks 1995). However, it is always worth remembering that pregnancy is the most common cause of secondary amenorrhoea.

Combined oral contraceptives will usually create a regular withdrawal bleed but all progestogen-only methods, whether administered as pills, implants, vaginal rings or depot injections, have poor cycle control. The levonorgestrel intrauterine system can also lead to irregular spotting and amenorrhoea. Bleeding irregularities may not be a great disadvantage, however, particularly in a woman who is used to oligomenorrhoea, as long as appropriate counselling is given prior to choosing the method.

Obesity

Obesity, defined as a body mass index (BMI) greater than 25 kg/m^2, is observed in about a third of women with PCOS (Polson et al. 1988). Obesity in women with PCOS is characterized by a fat distribution favouring the upper body segment (Bringer et al. 1994), with a waist/hip ratio of more than 0.85. This type of fat distribution is detected even in PCOS patients with a normal BMI.

Obesity has relevance to contraceptive use in a number of ways. It is the only risk factor for both arterial and venous disease and both these risks will be increased by the use of combined contraceptive preparations. Preparations containing the newer progestogens such as gestodene and desogestrel may have a greater effect on the risk of venous thrombosis but less of an effect on the risk of myocardial infarction in these patients.

Obese women who choose a levonorgestrel-releasing implant (Norplant) have a lower serum concentration of levonorgestrel (Sivin et al. 1997) and hence a greater contraceptive failure rate.

Sadly, the non-contraceptive effects of hormonal contraception tend to worsen rather than improve obesity. Weight gain is thought to result from the progestogen component of the combined oral contraceptive. This can be due to an increased appetite, in which case it usually responds to dietary restriction, or the anabolic effect of the progestogen. Pills containing desogestrel (Kaunitz 1993), gestodene (Ball et al. 1990) or norgestimate (Lippman 1992) do not appear to adversely effect weight gain. In women with PCOS, however, weight gain is unpredictable and the patient should be aware of this.

Obese women with PCOS run a variety of health risks as a direct result of their obesity: these include haemorrhoids, visceral hernias and osteoarthrosis. Despite the fact that many of these women have the greatest desire to lose weight it is extremely difficult to encourage successful weight loss in PCOS patients. Understandably, patients are unlikely to choose any form of contraception that they think might make them gain even a small amount of weight.

The syndrome is self-enhancing as oestrogens

are converted into androgens in peripheral adipose tissue. This probably explains why the severity of the symptoms has a tendency to increase with time.

Long-term health risks—and how contraceptive hormones may help

Hyperinsulinaemia

Women with PCOS may exhibit insulin resistance, particularly if they are anovulatory. However, the majority compensate by an increased pancreatic response to carbohydrate and so remain euglycaemic. Only a minority of young women with PCOS have mildly impaired glucose tolerance curves. A tendency to diabetes is revealed by drugs with an insulin antagonist action (Fox and Wardle 1990) but this does not include contraceptive steroids.

In a group of women with PCOS who conceived after ovarian electrodiathermy there was a 27-fold increase in gestational diabetes (Gjonnaess 1989). Long-term follow-up of women with PCOS has shown that at least 15% will develop frank diabetes by late middle age (Dahlgren et al. 1992).

Carbohydrate metabolism is only minimally affected by desogestrel (Shoupe 1993). Gestodene while having no impact on either lipid or carbohydrate metabolism did cause mild hyperinsulinism (Rabe et al. 1987). No adverse effects have been demonstrated in norgestimate-treated patients with respect to blood glucose or insulin concentrations (Burkman et al. 1992, Lippman 1992).

Hyperlipidaemia and coronary artery disease

Insulin is an important regulator of lipids and lipoproteins. It is therefore not surprising to find that patients with insulin resistance demonstrate lipid abnormalities. The overall prevalence of lipid abnormality in women with PCOS has been reported to be 80% in obese women, 39% in non-obese women and 10% in controls (Fox et al. 1991). In a group of women with PCOS who underwent suppression of steroidogenesis, the triglyceride level fell by 4% whilst the mean high-density lipoprotein C (HDL-C) level increased by 25% (Samra et al. 1989). The hypertriglyceridaemia is a direct result of the insulin resistance, whilst the disturbance in cholesterol metabolism is dependent on alteration in sex steroid concentration.

Eighty per cent of obese women with PCOS have lipid abnormality

There is also some epidemiological evidence to show an increased risk of cardiovascular

Table 2
Risk factors for arterial disease and venous thromboembolism.

Risk factors for arterial disease	Risk factors for venous thromboembolism
Family history	Obesity
Diabetes mellitus	Sedentary lifestyle
Hypertension	Inherited thrombophilia
Cigarette smoking	Severe varicose veins
Age	
Obesity	
Migraine	

disease in PCOS. Young women with coronary artery disease have been shown to have clinical sings of androgen excess (Wild et al. 1990). However, the degree of risk for cardiovascular disease in PCOS has yet to be quantified.

It is extremely important, from a contraceptive steroid point of view, to distinguish between venous and arterial disease. Patients at increased risk of venous thromboembolism (VTE) are rarely also at increased risk of myocardial infarction (MI) because the conditions have different aetiologies (*Table 2*). The exception is obese patients and these are discussed above. The classical view is that the oestrogen component of contraceptive agents increases the risk of VTE, whereas the androgenic progestogen component alters blood lipids so as to increase

the risk of MI. Hence the efforts of the pharmaceutical industry to produce less androgenic and more 'lipid friendly' progestogens. There is now much evidence to say that this view is far too simplistic. Most notably, combined oral contraceptive use has never been shown to produce atheroma or angina, or increase the risk of MI in past users. Nevertheless, modern progestogens may be preferable as they have a much more favourable effect on blood lipids (Zacur and Stewart 1992).

Desogestrel increases the concentration of high-density lipoproteins (HDL) and decreases that of low-density lipoproteins (LDL) (Burkman 1993). Gestodene increases triglyceride and phospholipid levels (Shoupe 1993) but the overall adverse effects when combined with ethinyloestradiol are minimal.

Norgestimate improves the lipid profile by increasing the HDL/LDL ratio (Burkman et al. 1992, Lippman 1992).

It seems reasonable to offer lipid screening to a woman with clinical features of PCOS, whether or not she is seeking help with contraception

A serum cholesterol concentration greater than 7.5 mmol/l is usually considered to be a contraindication to combined oral contraceptive use, although the level of risk is unknown. The concern here is not that the pill will increase the hyperlipidaemia (it may even lead to some improvement), but arteries with atheroma may be more susceptible to pill-induced thrombosis.

If combined oral contraception is felt to be the most appropriate contraceptive method for a PCOS patient, a balance needs to be considered between her risk of VTE and her risk of MI or stroke. If she is at greater risk of arterial disease a pill containing desogestrel, gestodene or norgestimate may be more appropriate because of their more favourable

effect on blood lipids. If she is at greater risk from VTE, a pill with an older progestogen such as levonorgestrel may be more appropriate because this may give less of an increase in her VTE risk. In general both these complications are rare, although arterial disease has the greater mortality and morbidity. Cigarette smoking and family history increase the risk of arterial disease.

It remains to be seen whether pills containing antiandrogenic progestogens will have a favourable effect of the lipid profile. Nomegesterol has been used in cases of type IIa dyslipoproteinaemia (Zartarian et al. 1998) (*Table 3*).

Endometrial and breast carcinoma

In anovulatory women with PCOS the oestrogenic affect on the uterus is unopposed by progesterone. This therefore increases the risk of endometrial hyperplasia, which can progress to carcinoma. A similar unopposed oestrogenic stimulation on breast tissue might be expected to have a similar oncogenic effect.

Any progestogen, whether given cyclically or continuously, will reduce the risk of endometrial hyperplasia. The levonorgestrel intrauterine contraceptive device delivers a high dose of progestogen to the endometrium and is probably a convenient way to reduce

Table 3
Androgenic effects of progestogens.

Progesterone	Antiandrogenic effects	Androgenic activity	Effect on SHBG
Gestodene	No	Weak[a]	Decreased[a]
Desogestrel	Reduced testosterone levels[b]	No	Decreased
Norgestimate	No[c]	Weak[c]	↔
Nomegestrol	Yes[d,e]	No[d,c]	↔
Dienogest	Yes[f]	No[f]	↔
Levonorgestrel	No	Yes	Decreased
Cyproterone	Yes	No	Decreased

[a]Kuhnz et al. (1992)
[b]Cullberg (1984)
[c]Halm et al. (1977)
[d]Botella et al. (1987)
[e]Paris et al (1983)
[f]Oettel et al. (1995)

the possibility of endometrial malignancy in these women. However, it is larger than other intrauterine devices and this may lead to an insertion problem in PCOS patients, many of whom are nulliparous.

The hyperandrogenism and hyperinsulinaemia of PCOS have prompted many researchers to suggest an association between PCOS and breast carcinoma (Kaaks 1996). Epidemiological evidence is, however, lacking (Anderson et al. 1997) and there is even some evidence that breast cancer rates are reduced in patients with PCOS (Gammon and Thompson 1992).

Conclusion

Asymptomatic women with the ultrasound diagnosis of polycystic ovaries (PCO) should be regarded as normal. Women with PCO and symptoms of hyperandrogenism or obesity or anovulation should be diagnosed as having polycystic ovary syndrome (PCOS).

Patients with PCOS, whether seeking contraceptive advice or not, should be aware of the genetic nature of their condition and their long-term health risks. These include cardiovascular disease, endometrial carcinoma and diabetes mellitus type II. If the patient can achieve weight loss this will alleviate many androgenic symptoms and reduce her risks of cardiovascular disease and diabetes. Serum lipid screening should be offered because modification of diet can improve future health.

A combined pill containing an antiandrogenic progestogen is the most effective at reducing symptoms of acne and hirsutism, but needs to be taken for more than 3 months

A combined preparation containing one of the antiandrogenic progestogens would appear to have the greatest non-contraceptive benefits for women with PCOS. By using such a pill a beneficial effect can be obtained for the androgenic symptoms, the risk of arterial disease and the risk of endometrial carcinoma. Similar benefits should be afforded by combined preparations delivered as monthly injectables or via an intravaginal ring.

Progestogen-only forms of contraception may reduce the risk of endometrial carcinoma.

Non-hormonal forms of contraception have no specific benefit or risk for women with PCOS.

It is particularly important to follow up women with PCOS who take combined oral contraception, not least because of their increased risk of hypertension and diabetes.

Case histories
Case 1

Sally, a 19-year-old female student, attends her general practitioner's surgery the week following a visit to the local accident and emergency department with an episode of lower abdominal pain. All investigations then had been negative, her symptoms had gradually subsided and she had been allowed home. No definite diagnosis has been made.

'I had an ultrasound scan which showed that I have polycystic ovaries, and I want to know what's wrong with me', she says.

Essential investigations by her general practitioner include a menstrual history, measurement of height, weight and blood pressure, and enquiries about family history, hair growth and acne. She does not consider herself hirsute and has a reasonably regular menstrual cycle of between 26 and 30 days. She uses condoms as she feels these are the 'safest' form of contraception. Her BMI is 22.

Sally needs much reassurance that polycystic ovaries are just a variant of normal and are of no relevance to her health. The conversation is switched to her reliance on condoms and the risk of contraceptive failure.

Case 2

Jean, a 26-year-old nurse, seeks her general practitioner's advice about contraception because her father has just had a heart attack at the age of 58. She has taken the combined pill for the past 18 months but is worried that because she is overweight and smokes it will increase her chances of cardiac disease in the future.

'Dad's attack made me think about things', she says.

Jean's BMI is 32 and she has some hair on her upper lip. Her periods when she is not taking the pill can be anything up to 6 weeks apart. There is no other family history of cardiac disease but she has one fat sister who is trying to get pregnant and one thin sister with two children.

Essential investigations are measurement of fasting serum cholesterol, which is 6.0 mmol/l, urinalysis, which is normal, and blood pressure, which is 130/80 mmHg. The diagnosis is PCOS. The genetics of her condition and the risks to her future health are explained to her. Having a definite diagnosis, she says, will help her to give up smoking, and she requests an ultrasound scan, which confirms the polycystic nature of her ovaries.

She has no major contraindication to the pill and is reassured, although she is advised strongly about her smoking and given an appointment to see the dietician.

References

Adams J, Franks S, Polson DW et al. (1985) Multifollicular ovaries: clinical and endocrine features and response to pulsatile gonadotrophin releasing hormone. *Lancet* ii: 1375–8.

Anderson KE, Sellers TA, Chen PL, Rich SS, Hong CP, Folsom AR (1997) Association of Stein–Leventhal syndrome with the incidence of postmenopausal breast cancer in a large prospective study of women in Iowa. *Cancer* 80(7): 1360–2.

Azziz R, Gay F (1989) The treatment of hyperandrogenism with oral contraceptives. *Semin Reprod Endocrin* 7: 246–54.

Balen AH, Conway GS, Kaltas G et al. (1995) Polycystic ovary syndrome: the spectrum of the disorder in 1741 patients. *Hum Reprod* 10: 2107–11.

Ball MJ, Ashwell E, Jackson M, Gillmer MDG (1990) Comparison of two triphasic contraceptives with different progestogens: effects on metabolism and coagulation proteins. *Contraception* 41: 363–76.

Botella J, Paris J, Lahlou B (1987) The cellular mechanism of the antiandrogenic action of nomegestrol acetate, a new 19-nor-progestagen on the rat prostate. *Acta Endocrinol* 115: 544–50.

Bringer J, Lefebvre P, Boulet F et al. (1994) Body composition and regional fat distribution in polycystic ovarian syndrome. Relationship to hormonal and metabolic profiles. *Ann NY Acad Sci* 687: 115–23.

Burkman RT (1993) Lipid metabolism effects with desogestrel-containing oral contraceptives. *Am J Obstet Gynecol* 168: 1033–40.

Burkman RT, Kafrissen ME, Olson W, Osterman J (1992) Lipid and carbohydrate effects of a new triphasic containing norgestimate. *Acta Obstet Gynaecol Scand* 71(suppl 156): 5–8.

Cullberg G (1984) Androgenic, anabolic, estrogenic and antiestrogenic effects of desogestrel and lynestrenol: effects on serum proteins and vaginal cytology. *Contraception* 30: 73–9.

Dahlgren E, Johansson S, Lindstedt G et al. (1992) Women with polycystic ovary syndrome wedge resected in 1956 to 1965: a long-term follow-up focusing on natural history and circulating hormones. *Fertil Steril* 57: 505–13.

Delahunt JW (1993) Hirsutism—practical therapeutic guidelines. *Drugs* 45: 223–31.

Ehrmann DA, Barnes RB, Rosenfield RL (1995) Polycystic ovary syndrome: a form of functional ovarian hyperandrogenism due to dysregulation of androgen secretion. *Endocr Rev* 16; 322–53.

Falsetti L, Galbignani E (1990) Long-term treatment with the combination ethinylestradiol and cyproterone acetate in polycystic ovary syndrome. *Contraception* 42(6): 611–19.

Fox R, Wardle PG (1990) Maturity-onset diabetes mellitus in association with polycystic ovarian disease and sex-steroid therapy. *J Obstet Gynaecol* 10: 555–6.

Fox R, Corrigan E, Coulson C, Hull MCR (1991) Studies of lipid state in polycystic ovarian disease. *Br J Obstet Gynaecol* 98: 1307.

Franks S (1995) Polycystic ovary syndrome. *New Engl J Med* 333: 856–61.

Gammon MD, Thompson WD (1992) Polycystic ovaries and the risk of breast cancer. *Am J Epidemiol* 136(3): 372–3.

Gjonnaess H (1989) The course and outcome of pregnancy after ovarian electrocautery in women with polycystic ovarian syndrome: the influence of body-weight. *Br J Obstet Gynaecol* 96: 714–19.

Gonzales CJ, Curson R, Parsons J (1988) Transabdominal versus transvaginal ultrasound screening of ovarian follicles: are they compatible? *Fertil Steril* 50: 657–9.

Guillebaud J (1995) Advising women on which pill to take. *Br Med J* 311: 1111–12.

Halm DW, Allen GO, McGuire JL (1977) The pharmacological profile of norgestimate, a new orally active progestin. *Contraception* 16: 541–53.

Kaaks R (1996) Nutrition, hormones, and breast cancer: is insulin the missing link? *Cancer Causes Contr* 7(6): 569–71.

Kaunitz AM (1993) Combined oral contraception with desogestrel/ethinyl oestradiol: tolerability profile. *Am J Obstet Gynecol* 168: 1028–33.

Kimura I, Togashi K, Kawakami S et al. (1996) Polycystic ovaries: implications of diagnosis with MR imaging. *Radiology* 210(2): 322–53.

Kuhnz W, Gansau C, Fuhrmeister A (1992) Pharmacokinetics of gestodene in 12 women who received a single oral dose of 0.075 mg gestodene and after a wash-out phase, the same dose during one treatment cycle. *Contraception* 46: 29–40.

Lippman J (1992) Long term profile of a new progestin. *Int J Fertil* 37(suppl 4): 218–22.

Mango D, Ricci S, Manna P, Miggiano GA, Serra GB (1996) Clinical and hormonal effects of ethinylestradiol combined with gestodene and desogestrel in young women with acne vulgaris. *Contraception* 53(3): 163–70.

McKenna TJ (1991) The use of anti-androgens in the treatment of hirsutism. *Clin Endocrinol* 35: 1–3.

Oettel M, Elger W, Ernst M et al. (1995) Experimentelle Endokrinpharmakologie von Dienogest. In: Tiechmann AT (ed.) *Dienogest-Präklinik und Klinik eines neuen Gestagens*, pp 11–21. Berlin: Walter de Gruyter Verlag.

Palatsi R, Hirvensalo E, Liukko P et al. (1984) Serum total and unbound testosterone and sex hormone-binding globulin (SHBG) in female acne patients treated with two different oral contraceptives. *Acta Derm Venereol (Stockh)* 64: 517–23.

Paris J, Thevenot R, Bonnet P et al. (1983) The pharmacological profile of TX 066 (17α-acetoxy-6-methyl-19-nor-4,6-pregnadiene-3,20-dione) a new oral progestative. *Drug Res* 33: 710–15.

Polson DW, Wadsworth J, Adams J, Franks S (1988) Polycystic ovaries: a common finding in normal women. *Lancet* i: 870–2.

Porcile A, Gallardo E (1991) Long term treatment of hirsutism: desogestrel compared with cyproterone acetate in oral contraceptives. *Fertil Steril* 55: 877–81.

Rabe T, Runnebaum B, Kohlmeier M, Harenberg J, Wiecher H, Unger R (1987) Clinical and metabolic effects of gestodene and levonorgestrel. *Int J Fertil* 32(suppl): 29–44.

Runnebaum B (1992) The androgenicity of oral contraceptives: the young patient's concerns. *Int J Fertil* 37(suppl 4): 211–17.

Samra JS, Brown P, Tang LC et al. (1989) Effects of medical oophorectomy on lipid profile in women with polycystic ovary syndrome. *J Endocrinol* 123(suppl): abstract 87.

Saxton DW, Farquar CM, Rae T, Beard RW, Anderson MC, Wadsworth J (1990) Accuracy of ultrasound measurement of female pelvic organs. *Br J Obstet Gynaecol* 97: 695–9.

Shoupe D (1993) Effects of desogestrel on carbohydrate metabolism. *Am J Obstet Gynecol* 168: 1041–7.

Sivin I, Lahteenmaki P, Ranta S et al. (1997) Levonorgestrel concentrations during use of levonorgestrel rod implants. *Contraception* 55: 81–5.

Stein IF, Leventhal ML (1935) Amenorrhoea associated with bilateral polycystic ovaries. *Am J Obstet Gynecol* 29: 181–91.

Swanson M, Sauerbrei EE, Cooperberg PL (1981) Medical implication of ultrasonically detected polycystic ovaries. *J Clin Ultrasound* 9: 219–22.

Wild RA, Grubb B, Hartz A, Van Nort JJ, Baghman W, Bartholomew M (1990) Clinical signs of androgen excess as risk factors for coronary artery disease. *Fertil Steril* 45: 255–9.

Zacur HA, Stewart D (1992) New concepts in oral contraceptive pill use. *Curr Opin Obstet Gynecol* 4: 365–71.

Zartarian M, Chevalier T, Micheletti MC, Leber C, Jamin C (1998) Biological and clinical safety of nomegestrol acetate administered alone then associated in inverse sequence with transdermal 17 beta estradiol, in women at risk of dyslipoproteinemia type IIa [French]. *Ann Endocrinol* 59(5): 411–16.

Women with cervical problems

Kay McAllister, Urszula Bankowska and Alison Bigrigg

9

Contraception and the cervical screening programme

The NHS cervical screening programme

Cervical screening has been shown to be, and is used as, an effective method of detecting precancerous changes within the cervix since the 1960s. During 1988, this became more organized with the introduction of the National Health Service cervical screening programme (NHSCSP). Each health authority was required to screen all women aged 20–64 years at least every 5 years, and to introduce a computerized call and recall system (NHSCSP 1996). This programme has resulted in a significant fall in both the incidence of and mortality from cervical cancer. In England and Wales, the incidence has fallen from 16.1 new cases per 100 000 women in 1986 to 11.2 per 100 000 in 1993, thus achieving several years ahead of schedule the government's *Health of the Nation* target of a 20% reduction by the year 2000 from the baseline figures of 1986. A comparable drop has also been seen in the Scottish figures.

Opportunistic screening

Smears may be offered opportunistically to women who fulfil the criteria of the NHSCSP, but who have failed to respond to the call and recall system. These women may be attending for other gynaecological or medical reasons, and the opportunity should be taken to enquire about their smear history during the consultation. There is no recommendation, and no justification, for performing smears in pregnancy, within 3 months postnatally or following termination, unless it is felt that this may be the only opportunity for the examination. Particular problems often arise in women from ethnic minorities, usually from a combination of religious and cultural beliefs.

Overscreening

Smears taken outwith the guidelines of the NHSCSP are not simply inappropriate clinically, but result in an increased financial and workload burden for those laboratories involved. Many clinicians are unaware of the screening programme guidelines, resulting in 'routine' unjustified smears (NHSCSP 1997). Within the family planning and community gynaecology setting, the following situations should *not* warrant an additional smear outwith the programme guidelines:

- on insertion of an intrauterine device (IUD) or hormone-releasing intrauterine system (IUS)

- while taking swabs to investigate vaginal discharge and/or infection

- in women with risk factors for cervical cancer, e.g. cigarette smokers, exposure to multiple sexual partners, presence of or history of genital warts or other sexually transmitted diseases

- as part of the investigation of abnormal vaginal bleeding, e.g. intermenstrual, postcoital.

It was also previous practice to repeat a smear 1 year following the initial smear in the programme. This has also been shown to be unnecessary.

There is no justification for offering cervical smears to sexually active teenagers

The first smear should be offered after a woman's twentieth birthday and may be delayed to the second or subsequent consultations concerning contraception.

Screening at first visit

This situation is most frequently encountered when a young girl presents for contraceptive advice. Again, previous standard practice was to offer a smear at this point. Following the 1992 guidelines from the NHSCSP, the routine taking of smears in those under the age of 20 years is not recommended. The rationale behind this lies in the 1996 figures for England and Wales, which show no deaths in teenagers from cervical cancer, although teenagers may develop cervical intraepithelial neoplasia (CIN).

The call and recall system is initiated at age 20 years, but need not result in an immediate smear. Provided one is obtained within the next 4–5 years, no urgency or undue pressure should be placed on the women before this (Cuzick et al. 1998). Many clinics prefer to defer the first examination until the second or subsequent consultation concerning contraception, even in a 20-year-old. This is wholly appropriate, as the patient has a great deal of information to absorb at the first visit and the clinician is aiming to put her at as much ease as possible. There is also the possible disadvantage of unnecessary intervention for minor cervical changes, many of which often revert to normal spontaneously. There is also the danger of complications such as cervical stenosis or haemorrhage after treatment.

Associated risk of CIN with different types of contraception

Many epidemiological studies have investigated the association between contraception and the risk of developing CIN. Common to the majority of studies is the difficulty in excluding other variables which are generally accepted to have contributory effects on the cervix. These include age at first coitus, number of sexual partners, smoking, immunological status and infections including chlamydia and human papillomavirus (HPV) (Etherington and Shaf 1996).

However, there is reasonable evidence to suggest the effects on the cervix of each type of contraception.

Condoms

Condoms offer protection, if used correctly, against sexually transmitted diseases, including human immunodeficiency virus (HIV). They will also reduce the incidence of virus-induced or associated cervical changes, including herpes simplex and HPV. The relative risk of severe dysplasia after 10 years use is 0.2 compared with 4.0 for combined oral contraceptive users (Kirkman 1993).

Diaphragms

The physical nature of this method results in cervical protection similar to that of condom use. However, this may also reflect the associated lifestyle of the diaphragm users, which is in general more stable than the average patient.

COCs

All studies suggest that sexual lifestyle is far more indicative of risk than combined oral contraceptive (COC) use *per se*. The primary cofactor is undoubtedly sexually transmitted, with HPV at present the most common link. However, if these variables are not taken into consideration there is suggestion of up to 50% increased risk of squamous cell carcinoma and a doubled risk of the less common adenocarcinoma (Ursin et al. 1995).

Progestogen-only pill

No association has been found with either an increased or decreased risk of CIN developing amongst progestogen-only pill (POP) users (McCann and Potter 1994).

Depot medroxyprogesterone acetate

There has been no proven risk associated with depot medroxyprogesterone acetate. Any small association is suspected to be due to confounding factors, especially smoking and sexual activity.

IUDs

There is no known effect other than those associated with lifestyle (Farley et al. 1992). There are no overall health benefits of IUDs other than decreasing the chance of pregnancy. They neither protect from nor increase the incidence of pelvic infection.

Benign cervical conditions

Benign cervical conditions can give rise to symptoms of intermenstrual bleeding, postcoital bleeding and excessive vaginal discharge. If a patient complains of these symptoms, a speculum examination should be performed to exclude a physical cause. It is not necessary to perform a cervical smear as CIN does not give rise to these symptoms. Any cervical appearance suggestive of cervical malignancy needs urgent referral for colposcopic assessment and biopsy.

Cervical smears taken outwith the screening programme are not justified in patients during or 3 months after pregnancy, prior to insertion of an IUD or IUS, or during investigations for infection or abnormal bleeding.

A cervical smear is only justified if pre-invasive neoplasia needs to be excluded

Cervical ectopy

Ectopy, often incorrectly referred to as erosion of the cervix, is a benign condition which occurs when columnar epithelium, normally present in the endocervix, everts and is found on the ectocervix. This results in a red and occasionally friable cervix, as the more vascular endocervical stroma is seen through the thinner endocervical epithelium.

The majority of cases are asymptomatic, but there may be excessive vaginal discharge or contact bleeding, noticeable as postcoital bleeding or after a smear has been taken. Ectopy is not an abnormal finding, and unless producing troublesome symptoms does not require treatment. More marked ectopy can be seen at other times, for example during pregnancy. During this time, the increased circulating hormone levels stimulate eversion. A similar effect is noted in users of the combined oral contraceptive pill. If symptoms remain troublesome, treatment options include cryocautery or cold coagulation. It is important to ensure there is a normal smear history before any cervical treatments.

Cervical polyps

The majority of cervical polyps are asymptomatic and are regarded by many as a normal finding. They are extremely common and typically arise from endocervical columnar epithelium. If large enough, they may present through the external os. They are usually soft and frequently show surface ulceration. There may be an associated inflammatory reaction with squamous metaplasia of the columnar epithelium. There is no association with malignant change, although the appearance may mimic squamous cell carcinoma. A polyp may also be mistaken for a submucous fibroid, which has developed a stalk and protruded through the os.

Polyps may cause irregular bleeding, especially if the surface is necrotic. In these cases, removal is curative. The entire polyp, including stalk down to the base, must be excised to prevent regrowth. If the base can be seen clearly, this is easily performed as an outpatient procedure using simple polyp forceps to grasp the base. The entire specimen can be twisted off, with no need for local anaesthesia. If the base cannot be identified, hysteroscopy is often a helpful aid. There is no known association between any form of contraception and the development of cervical polyps.

Abnormal bleeding may result from cervical ectopy, polyps, inflammatory changes or neoplasia. Whilst CIN does not result in abnormal bleeding, it may coexist with these causes.

CIN does not result in abnormal bleeding

Inflammatory changes

Inflammation of the cervix is common and in itself is of little significance. Inflammatory damage may arise from a variety of stimuli, including infection and trauma. The end result is often noted in smear reports when metaplastic cells are seen. However, this can with inexperience be confused with cervical neoplasia.

Acute inflammation produces numerous polymorphonuclear leucocytes, which can be seen as an inflammatory exudate on the smear sample. Ectopy, pregnancy and the COC may also produce this appearance. In chronic inflammation, lymphocytes are an additional feature. It is important to determine whether dyskaryosis is present; if not, there is no justification for an early repeat smear.

Changes associated with combined oral contraception

Cervical smears from women using the COC range from atrophic patterns to a well-oestrogenized pattern with predominantly superficial squamous cells. Unsatisfactory smears may arise as an effect of the COC owing to excessive clumping and folding of cells and large numbers of Döderlein's bacilli.

At colposcopic examination the cervix will often be enlarged and hyperaemic. The squamous epithelium is unaffected but changes are recognized in the columnar epithelium with enlargement and hyperaemia occurring in normal villi (Critchlow et al. 1995). This may give an almost polypoid appearance. Histologically, this may be associated with microglandular endocervical hyperplasia; this is a combination of cellular changes in the endocervix resulting from progestogenic influences on the epithelium, commonly seen in women taking the COC and in pregnancy and also reported in postmenopausal women. Usually the cervix is microscopically normal, but occasionally microglandular endocervical hyperplasia is so florid that it presents as cervical polyps visible to the naked eye.

Influences on contraceptive choice

Women base their decisions on contraception choice on many factors. There is a need to balance contraceptive efficacy with acceptability of method and health risks and benefits. In asymptomatic women the presence of benign cervical conditions need not be a factor in influencing contraceptive choice. A number of studies have suggested that cervical ectopy enhances the susceptibility of the cervix to infection by *Chlamydia trachomatis*. Women should be counselled with regard to good sexual health practices and the benefits of using a barrier method of contraception in addition to a hormonal method of contraception at risk times for infection.

Cervical intraepithelial neoplasia

Contraception during colposcopic surveillance or treatment

As discussed earlier, contraception has little or no effect on CIN compared with sexual lifestyle as a whole, with the exception of barrier methods. Prior to and during treatment, the woman's contraception needs should be discussed. Unless there are other reasons for doing so, oral contraception should be continued as usual. If a monophasic pill is used, two packets run consecutively may avoid a withdrawal bleed if this coincides with the colposcopy appointment, and may minimize bleeding after treatment. This, of course, is not the case with progestogen-only pills. Indeed, as colposcopy treatment often involves ablative therapy, the destruction of mucus-secreting glands may theoretically render the pill temporarily less efficient

following treatment, although there is no evidence to support this.

The obvious problem relates to IUD users. If colposcopy alone is performed, the threads can simply be moved to allow a clear view of the squamocolumnar junction. Similarly, a punch biopsy should not pose a problem. However, if large loop excision of the transformation zone (LLETZ) is necessary, it is recommended that the device is removed because the electric loop would cut through the threads making future removal difficult.

Following an abnormal smear

There is no absolute need or indication for contraception to be changed following an abnormal smear. It is much better to continue an established method than increase the risk of unplanned pregnancy. The opportunity should be taken, however, to explain to the woman the beneficial effects of barrier methods of contraception.

Actinomycosis

The genus *Actinomyces* consists of several species of Gram-positive bacteria with a tendency to form branching filaments. They form part of the normal flora of the oral cavity and bowel, but take advantage of infection, trauma or surgical injury to penetrate normally intact mucosal barriers. Actinomycetes have been found to be present at the cervix as a commensal in 1–5% of women.

Not all *Actinomyces*-like organisms reported cytologically represent true *Actinomyces* infection. The policy is one of actively monitoring for symptoms rather than unnecessary interventions in asymptomatic women.

The presence of Actinomyces-like organisms does not necessarily demand treatment

The presence of *Actinomyces*-like organisms (ALOs) may be noted on cervical smears of IUD or IUS users. This does not necessarily represent a pathological state, as it may occur in asymptomatic women. The overall risk of developing an *Actinomyces* infection with an IUD or IUS is extremely small, but prolonged use of an IUD, associated with stubborn or recurrent pelvic infection, should alert the clinician to the possibility. All women with ALOs reported on a smear should be given information with regard to this and management options discussed with them. In asymptomatic women, the choices are either to leave the IUD *in situ*, with careful follow-up, or to remove the device, with or without insertion of a new device at the same consultation.

When the device is left *in situ*, follow-up must include regular examinations, with careful attention to specific symptoms. It is generally regarded as reasonable that these checks should be 6-monthly. Cervical smears should continue to be checked according to screening guidelines. The woman should be asked specifically about any vaginal discharge, deep dyspareunia, pelvic pain, fever or intermenstrual bleeding. Should these occur, she should be aware of the necessity to seek medical advice promptly.

When the device is removed without another being inserted, the cytological findings will usually revert to normal within 8–12 weeks. In these cases there is no need for antibiotic treatment as this represents superficial colonization by these commensals, rather than any pathological state of the cervix.

In the presence of symptoms, or in women for whom pelvic infection is suspected, removal of the device is recommended. Whilst this condition may only consist of vaginal discharge, in some women it can progress to severe pelvic inflammatory disease with abscess formation and all the problems following this (Burkman et al. 1982). The device, with threads excised, should be sent for bacteriological culture with a specific request to look for *Actinomyces*. An endocervical swab should be taken and sent at the same time. Treatment with high-dose, long-term penicillin should be commenced as soon as possible. When removing a device during the second half of the menstrual cycle, it should be remembered that any intercourse during the previous week may result in pregnancy. An alternative form of contraception should be arranged.

Case histories

Case 1

Kate, a 28-year-old woman has been using combined oral contraception for 3 years. She presents with intermenstrual spotting which is presumed to be breakthrough bleeding. Her pill is changed to a different preparation. Three months later, it has not settled. A further change is made. After 4 months her bleeding has not responded, so she is prescribed a triphasic pill to see if it helps. After a further 4 months, a speculum examination is performed and a fleshy cervical polyp noted. Following its avulsion, her intermenstrual bleeding settles. Histology is totally benign.

Case 2

Caroline, a 38-year-old woman with two children attends for her routine smear test. Her family is complete and she has an IUD in place. Her smear reports show moderate dyskaryosis. At colposcopy, extensive aceto-white changes are noted. Her IUD is removed and a LLETZ performed. Following this, she has vaginal staining for 4–5 weeks. When she returns for review 4 months later she has had no further bleeding and a pregnancy test is positive. She was found to be 12 weeks pregnant. She was unaware that conception could occur during the period of vaginal bleeding following her LLETZ.

References

Burkman R, Schlesselman S, McCaffrey L et al. (1982) The relationship of genital tract actinomycetes and the development of pelvic inflammatory disease. *Am J Obstet Gynecol* 143: 585–9.

Critchlow CW, Vulner-Hanssen P, Eschenbach DA et al. (1995) Determinance of cervical ectopia and of cervicitis: age, oral contraception, specific cervical infection, smoking and douching. *Am J Obstet Gynecol* 173: 534–43.

Cuzick J, Meijer CJLM, Walboomers JMM (1988) Screening for cervical cancer. *Lancet* 351: 1439–40.

Etherington IJ, Shafi MI (1996) Human papillomavirus testing in primary cervical screening. *Genitourin Med* 72: 153–4.

Farley TMM, Rosenberg MJ, Rowe PJ et al. (1992) IUDs and PID: perspectives from a large international data base. *Lancet* 39: 785–8.

Kirkman R (1993) Contraception and the prevention of STD. *Br Med Bull* 49: 171–81.

McCann MF, Potter LS (1994) Progestin-only oral contraception: a comprehensive review. *Contraception* 50: 193–5.

NHSCSP (1996) *Quality Assurance Guidelines for the Cervical Screening Programme. Report of a Working Party Convened by the NHS Cervical Screening Programme.* National Health Service Cervical Screening Programme publication no. 3.

NHSCSP (1997) *Guidelines for Clinical Practice and Programme Management,* 2nd edn. National Health Service Cervical Screening Programme publication no. 8.

Ursin G, Peters RK, Henderson BE et al. (1995) Oral contraceptive use and adenocarcinoma of cervix. *Lancet* 344: 1390–4.

Women with menorrhagia

Stephen Killick

Menorrhagia is common, has a profound influence on quality of life, and can be alleviated or exaggerated by the non-contraceptive effects of various contraceptive agents. Therefore heaviness of bleeding always has an important influence on contraceptive choice.

Epidemiology of menorrhagia

Troublesome symptoms related to menstruation are a relatively modern phenomenon. In times past women experienced a later menarche, a greater number of pregnancies and longer duration of breastfeeding episodes, which all combined to create a total life-long expectancy of only about 40 menstrual periods. Contemporary women now expect about 400 periods in their lifetime.

The term 'menorrhagia' should be used specifically for menstruation that is both heavy and regular. This is because the regularity of bleeding is determined by different factors from those that affect the heaviness of bleeding. Irregular bleeding is caused by abnormal hormone production or by bleeding from non-hormone-dependent tissue, neither of which cause a regular monthly blood loss. Menorrhagia, on the other hand, is associated with normal endometrial histology and normal cyclical sex hormone production.

A monthly blood loss of 80 ml or greater has been chosen as the objective definition of true menorrhagia following a Swedish population study (Hallberg et al. 1966). In this study 476 Swedish women were selected at random to have their menstrual blood loss measured objectively together with haematological assessments of iron storage. Mean monthly loss was found to be 43 ± 2.3 ml. Mean haemoglobin levels were lower in women with a monthly blood loss greater than 60 ml, and where losses exceeded 80 ml total iron binding capacity and iron stores were much reduced. The diagnostic cut-off of 80 ml was chosen as a level above which iron deficiency anaemia became increasingly probable.

Mean menstrual loss is about 40 ml a month

In European population studies about 20% of women have been shown to have a blood loss greater than 60 ml and about 10% have true menorrhagia (Cole et al. 1971, Rybo 1982).

Menstrual loss increases with parity and age. One study investigated the same group of 33 women at ages 38, 44 and 50 years (Rybo et al. 1985). Their mean loss doubled over this 12-year period, the greatest increase being in the second 6 years. Much of this increase might be due to the development of uterine fibroids, which are extremely common in women in their mid-forties.

Race is also relevant. Black women have a higher incidence of uterine fibroids and therefore a greater chance of developing menorrhagia. Chinese women have been shown to have a higher mean menstrual loss than European women (Goa et al. 1987).

Women who complain of heavy periods often state that their mother or their sister suffered similar problems. However, there is little objective evidence to support a strong genetic predisposition. Monozygotic twins have similar menstrual losses, but there is a poor correlation between the menstrual loss of dizygotic twins (Rybo and Hallberg 1966).

Diagnosis

Objective menstrual assessment requires the collection of the woman's entire used sanitary wear, to which large volumes of sodium hydroxide are added to produce alkaline haematin from the contained haemoglobin. The solution is then submitted to spectophotometry and the resulting extinction is proportional to the original volume of haemoglobin. This, as one can imagine, is a messy and somewhat hazardous process even in a research environment and is never used clinically. Objective assessment of menstrual loss is probably not relevant anyway because what really matters is a woman's subjective perception of her heaviness and whether this is a problem for her.

A woman's assessment of her own menstrual loss is notoriously poor. As many as 26% of women with normal blood loss consider their periods to be heavy, and 40% of those with objective menorrhagia consider their periods to be moderate or light (Hallberg et al. 1966). After all, a woman only has her own previous menstrual loss for comparison. If she has a usual loss of 30 ml a month and something happens to increase this to 60 ml (such as discontinuing oral contraception) she has experienced a 100% increase, which may or may not affect her life, but she still does not have true menorrhagia.

About a third of women, when surveyed for a MORI poll, said their periods had been heavy at some time, but only one third of these women had sought medical advice for the problem (Corrado 1990). There is, therefore, a large group of women who believe they have heavy periods and who would presumably wish their contraceptive method to be of some help, or at least not make things worse. Even women who do not consider their periods to be heavy often would prefer them to be

lighter. Conversely, there are many women who are not aware of the fact that their bleeding is pathologically heavy. Fitting a copper intrauterine device in such a woman may lead to bleeding heavy enough to cause iron deficiency anaemia.

Ten per cent of women suffer with true menorrhagia but a further 25% of women with normal loss believe they have heavy periods

There are a number of ways in which menstrual flow can be assessed by the clinical history. Women who bleed for more than 7 days have a mean loss of greater than 80 ml even though 86% of the total is lost in the first 3 days (Hallberg et al. 1966). The number of tampons or pads used is notoriously unreliable both because of the different absorbencies of different products and because women change their sanitary wear at different saturations. A tampon can hold up to 50 ml of blood but is often changed when it contains less than 10 ml.

Menorrhagia is certainly perceived to be a distressing symptom by those who seek medical help. A study by Coulter and her colleagues (Coulter et al. 1994) highlighted the associated features of moodiness and irritability (68%), depression (50%), interference with sex life (44%) or interference with life in general. Menorrhagia has particular problems for women with severe learning disabilities (see Chapter 14).

The large number of hysterectomies performed annually in the western world indicates how serious a problem heavy bleeding is viewed to be by the sufferer. In the USA 600 000 women undergo hysterectomy every year (6 per 1000), mainly for bleeding problems (Lepine et al. 1997).

Causes of menorrhagia—and their relevance to contraceptive methods

Fibroids

Uterine fibroids (myomata, leiomyomata) are extremely common. Their reported incidence varies according to the method used for their detection, although they are undoubtedly the most common single cause of menorrhagia. They can be detected in up to 77% of uteri if hysterectomy specimens are sectioned into 2 mm slices (Cramer and Patel 1990) and are also present in 50% of the general female population as noted post mortem (Wallach 1992). These figures qualify fibroids as the most common tumour seen in women of

reproductive age and probably the most common of all human tumours. Prehysterectomy diagnosis does not, of course, detect the majority of uteri with small and possibly clinically insignificant fibroids. Clinical examination will only reveal significantly enlarged or irregular uteri and then only in women who are thin enough to enable a meaningful bimanual examination to be performed. The accuracy of clinical diagnosis is poor and can lead to both under- and overdiagnosis (Cramer and Patel 1990). Vaginal ultrasonography will increase the likelihood of fibroid detection and has the added advantage of being able to localize the fibroids into submucous, interstitial or subserous varieties.

Fibroids may not only give rise to heavy periods. They have been implicated in a variety of other problems such as subfertility, recurrent miscarriage, pelvic pain, dysmenorrhoea and symptoms resulting from sheer size and pressure within the pelvis such as urinary frequency or a palpable pelvic mass. As with all associations between a common pathological feature and common symptoms, it is often unclear which—if any—of the symptoms a woman may complain of are truly the consequence of her fibroids or whether their presence is merely incidental.

The incidence of fibroids is influenced by a number of factors (*Table 1*). Fibroids are

Table 1
Factors influencing the incidence of uterine fibroids

Increased by	Decreased by
Age	Subfertility
Parity	Late menarche
Obesity	Cigarette smoking
Women of black African descent	Delayed birth of first child
	Combined oral contraception

oestrogen-dependent, and the effect of obesity and of smoking on oestrogen levels is thought to explain why the incidence of fibroids increases by 21% for every 10 kg increase in weight (Ross et al. 1986) and why smokers are less likely to develop fibroids than non-smokers. Combined oral contraception, for whatever reason, appears to be protective. The Oxford Family Planning Association study examined a cohort of 535 women who developed fibroids and matched them to controls. The incidence of fibroids was reduced by 31% after 10 years of oral contraceptive use (Ross et al. 1986). This effect on the prevalence of fibroids may be of minor clinical significance but combined oral contraception is an excellent treatment for the resulting menorrhagia (see below).

The effect of contraceptive steroids on existing fibroids is variable and unpredictable with the rare exception of the haemorrhagic cellular leiomyoma, which is stimulated by both oral contraception and pregnancy (Norris et al. 1988). Depot medroxyprogesterone acetate has been shown to increase the mitotic rate of fibroid tumours (Tiltman 1985) but this seems to have little effect on their growth.

Intrauterine contraceptive devices (IUCDs) are generally contraindicated for the woman with fibroids, for a number of reasons. Apart from the increase in menstrual loss associated with IUCD use, the device may be difficult to fit in an irregular endometrial cavity, and subsequent expulsion, discontinuation and pregnancy rates are much increased (*Figure 1*). Multiple small fibroids are probably irrelevant and a bimanual examination is usually thought adequate for determining whether an IUCD could be fitted or not. Occasionally a cavity may be felt to be irregular at insertion into what is thought to be a normal-sized uterus. In this case vaginal ultrasonography will usually demonstrate a submucous or polypoid lesion.

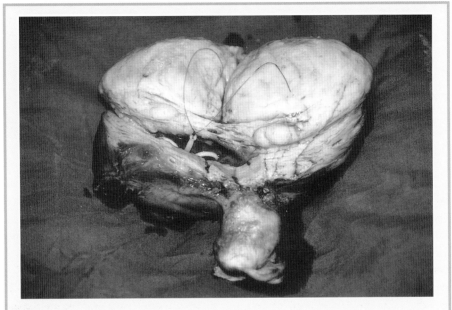

Figure 1
Hysterectomy specimen showing how a large fundal fibroid can distort the uterine cavity and dislodge an IUCD. In this case the fibroid, together with the symptom of menorrhagia, developed several years after the insertion of the device.

Idiopathic menorrhagia

When large fibroids have been excluded by bimanual examination menorrhagia may be the result of adenomyosis, multiple small fibroids or disordered prostaglandin metabolism within the uterine wall. More specific diagnosis is, however, clinically unhelpful, and the term 'idiopathic menorrhagia' is used pragmatically. In these cases a balance needs to be sought between the advantages and disadvantages of therapy, and appropriate management is usually arrived at by a stepwise approach (*Figure 2*). Careful reassurance may be all that is necessary after excluding gross uterine pathology and anaemia.

Non-steroidal analgesics and antifibrinolytic agents will treat menorrhagia but the reduction in menstrual loss is proportional to the excess over normal, so women who do not

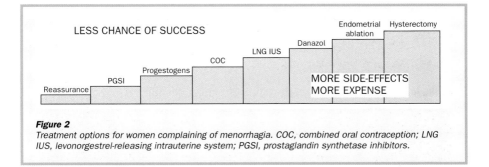

Figure 2
Treatment options for women complaining of menorrhagia. COC, combined oral contraception; LNG IUS, levonorgestrel-releasing intrauterine system; PGSI, prostaglandin synthetase inhibitors.

have high losses experience little benefit. There is also unlikely to be a reduction in the number of days of bleeding.

Combined oral contraception reduces menstrual loss in virtually all women. A measured reduction in mean blood loss from 60.2 ml to 36.5 ml was seen after 3 months of therapy with a pill containing 30 µg ethinyloestradiol and 150 µg gestodene (Larsson et al. 1992). The five women in this study who had true menorrhagia had their losses returned to normal and the low iron stores seen in two cases improved. An added advantage is that bleeding becomes predictable and of a shorter duration.

Cyclical progestogen therapy in which tablets are taken during the 10 days prior to menstruation is really only useful in cases of anovulation when a heavy, irregular bleeding pattern can be regulated. More prolonged administration of progestogens, when

ovulation is inhibited, is more useful for menorrhagia (Irvine et al. 1998) and most forms of progestogenic contraception can be used to lessen the menstrual loss. Progestogen-only pills, depot injections and subcutaneous rods all commonly reduce total menstrual loss, although bleeding can become irregular and unpredictable and the number of days on which bleeding occurs is often increased.

The levonorgestrel intrauterine system (IUS) is a relatively new treatment for menorrhagia and does not hold a licence for use other than for contraception in many countries. Nevertheless, the 20 µg of levonorgestrel released from the device daily has a profound effect on blood loss. Tissue levels of levonorgestrel are many times those achieved by oral administration and the endometrium quickly becomes atrophic with very few receptors for either oestrogen or progesterone. Serum hormone levels are unaltered in levonorgestrel IUS users and the effect on blood loss is exclusively local.

The levonorgestrel IUS reduces menstrual loss by 95%

The reduction in menstrual loss reaches 54% in the first month after insertion, 87% after 3 months and 95% after 6 months (Tang and Lo 1995). As many as 30% of women may become amenorrhoeic with prolonged use. The disadvantage, as with all other forms of exclusively progestogenic contraception, is that bleeding patterns are often irregular and spotting is common (Andersson and Rybo 1990). The total number of days a month on which bleeding or spotting occurs is usually increased by about 4 days during the first 3 months of use, and women should be fully informed of what to expect prior to insertion so as to avoid high removal rates.

Danazol is not an effective contraceptive and its androgenicity makes additional contraceptive precautions essential for fear of teratogenicity, although this appears to be more theoretical than real.

Hysterectomy is, of course, not only a 100% effective treatment for menorrhagia, whatever the aetiology, but also 100% effective contraception.

IUCD-induced menorrhagia

Non-medicated IUCDs are well known to increase both the duration and the heaviness of the menstrual flow. Generally speaking the greater the surface area of the IUCD the lower the contraceptive failure rate, but the greater the unwanted effects of menorrhagia, dysmenorrhoea and expulsion. Blood loss has been shown to increase by about 20 ml a month with modern copper devices (Larsson et al. 1975). It is interesting to note, however, that the women who had menorrhagia prior to insertion in this study did not experience an increase in their blood loss. Makarainen and Ylikorkala (1986) also measured an increase in menstrual loss of 74% after copper IUCD insertion but showed that this could be prevented by the prostaglandin synthetase inhibitor ibuprofen.

IUCD-induced menorrhagia can be reduced by prostaglandin synthetase inhibitors

Coagulation problems

Women who are anticoagulated virtually always have heavy periods and, by virtue of the reason for their anticoagulant therapy, a strong medical reason to avoid pregnancy. An example is women who are at risk of thromboembolic disease, for whom combined oral contraception is contraindicated. Barrier methods have a lower efficacy and intramuscular injections can cause severe bruising, so progestogens given either orally or by an intrauterine system are the methods of choice.

One particularly difficult problem is that of patients receiving haemodialysis who are not only anticoagulated but attached to a dialysis machine for long periods up to three times a week, making personal hygiene difficult. Although there is little need for contraception in this group, because dialysis leaches out sex hormones, the insertion of a levonorgestrel IUS can be very useful.

Sterilization

The vast majority of women who undergo sterilization do not experience a change in menstrual pattern, and even if they do it is most commonly attributable to the cessation of contraceptive methods which affect menstrual flow such as an IUCD or combined oral contraception (Bhiwandiwala et al. 1983). However, a large number of epidemiological studies have demonstrated an increased hysterectomy rate for menstrual disorders in women who have undergone sterilization. Typically the relative risk is about 1.9, but it is greater in younger women sterilized more

than 7 years previously (Goldhaber et al. 1993).

Sterilized women may, of course, be more willing to forgo their uterus as treatment for menstrual problems than women who have retained their fertility. In support of this argument, prospective studies have failed to show an increase in the menstrual dysfunction rate compared with controls (Rulin et al. 1993), and objective assessments of menstrual loss have not shown any effect of sterilization within 1 year (Sahwi et al. 1989).

There may be a physiological mechanism whereby sterilization might lead to disordered menstruation. Surgical disruption of the periovarian vasculature may interefere with hormone production. Endometrial microvascular perfusion has been shown to increase after sterilization (Verco et al. 1998).

A review of more than 200 articles (Gentile et al. 1998) has concluded that sterilization of women aged over 30 years does not increase the risk of menstrual dysfunction. There may, however, be an increased risk for women sterilized at a younger age.

Case histories

Case 1

Jenny, a 39-year-old woman, presents with a 2-year history of gradually increasing menorrhagia. She attributes her troubles to her laparoscopic sterilization procedure performed 2 years ago.

'I wish I had never had the operation,' she says. 'Nobody told me it could lead to this.'

A careful history reveals that she had taken combined oral contraception for 6 years prior to her operation. She is recently divorced and in a new relationship. She has also gone back to work after many years of staying at home with the family. She still bleeds for 5 days regularly each month but her tampon use has increased a little.

A pelvic examination is normal and she is not anaemic or clinically myxoedematous. It would appear that her natural increase in menstrual flow as she ages has been exaggerated by her intolerance because of her changed lifestyle.

She is reassured and given naproxen 500 mg twice daily to take from the day before menstruation, but returns in only 1 month saying the drug had no effect. She is then referred for endometrial resection.

Case 2

Rebecca, a mother of two, attends with her youngest daughter of 6 months requesting the insertion of an IUCD. When questioned she says her periods last for 8 or 9 days.

'They're certainly heavier than they used to be but they're no problem. I suppose that always happens when you have kids.'

Physical examination is normal but her haemoglobin level is 10.1 g/dl and the film shows an iron deficient picture.

She is still keen on an IUCD so is fitted with a levonorgestrel IUS after careful counselling about the probable irregularity of bleeding for the first few months.

References

Andersson JK, Rybo G (1990) Levonorgestrel releasing intrauterine device in the treatment of menorrhagia. *Br J Obstet Gynaecol* **97**: 690–4.

Bhiwandiwala PP, Mumford SD, Feldblum PJ (1983) Menstrual pattern changes following laparoscopic sterilisation with different occlusion techniques: a review of 10,004 cases. *Am J Obstet Gynecol* 145(6): 684–94.

Cole SK, Billewicz WZ, Thomson AM (1971) Sources of variation in menstrual blood loss. *J Obstet Gynaecol Br Com* **78**: 933–9.

Corrado M (1990) *Women's Health in 1990.* London: MORI.

Coulter A, Peto V, Jenkinson C (1994) Quality of life and patient satisfaction after treatment for menorrhagia. *Fam Pract* **11**: 394–401.

Cramer SF, Patel A (1990) The frequency of uterine leiomyomas. *Am J Clin Pathol* **94**: 435–9.

Gentile GP, Kaufman SC, Helbig DW (1998) Is there any evidence for a post-tubal sterilization syndrome? *Fertil Steril* **69**(2): 179–86.

Goa J, Zeng S, Sun BL et al. (1987) Menstrual bloodloss and haematological indices in healthy Chinese women. *J Reprod Med* **22**: 822–6.

Goldhaber MK, Armstrong MA, Golditch IM, Sheehe PR, Petitti DB, Friedman GD (1993) Long-term risk of hysterectomy among 80,007 sterilised and comparison women at Kaiser Permanente, 1971–1987. *Am J Epidemiol* **138**(7): 508–21.

Hallberg L, Hogdahl AM, Nilsson L, Rybo G (1966) Menstrual blood loss—a population study. *Acta Obstet Gynaecol Scand* **45**: 320–51.

Irvine GA, Campbell-Brown MB, Lumsden MA, Heikkila A, Walker JJ, Cameron IT (1998) Randomised comparative trial of the levonorgestrel intrauterine system and norethisterone for treatment of idiopathic menorrhagia. *Br J Obstet Gynaecol* **105**(6): 592–8.

Larsson B, Hamberger L, Rybo G (1975) Influence of copper intrauterine devices (Cu-7-IUD) on the menstrual bloodloss. *Acta Obstet Gynaecol Scand* **54**(4): 315–18.

Larsson G, Milsom I, Lindstedt G, Rybo (1992) The influence of a low dose combined oral contraceptive on menstrual blood loss and iron status. *Contraception* **46**(4): 327–34.

Lepine LA, Hills SD, Marchbanks PA et al. (1997) Hysterectomy surveillance–United States, 1980–1993. *MMWR CDC Surveillance Summaries* **46**(4): 1–15.

Makarainen L, Ylikorkala O (1986) Ibuprofen prevents IUCD-induced increases in menstrual blood loss. *Br J Obstet Gynaecol* **93**(3): 285–8.

Norris HJ, Hilliard GD, Irey NS (1988) Haemorrhagic cellular leiomyomas of the uterus associated with pregnancy and oral contraceptives. *Int J Gynecol Pathol* **7**(3): 212–24.

Ross RK, Pike MC, Vessey MP, Bull D, Yeates D, Casagrande JT (1986) Risk factors for uterine fibroids: reduced risk associated with oral contraceptives. *Br Med J Clin Res Ed* **293**(6543): 359–62.

Rybo G (1982) Population studies of menorrhagia. *Res Clin Forum* **4**: 77–81.

Rybo G, Hallberg L (1966) Influence of heredity and environment on normal menstrual blood loss. *Acta Obstet Gynaecol Scand* **45**: 57–79.

Rybo G, Leman J, Tibblin E (1985) Epidemiology of menstrual bloodloss. *Serono Symposia Publ.* Geneva: Serono. **25**: 181–93.

Rulin MC, Davidson AR, Philliber SG, Graves WL, Cushman LF (1993) Long term effects of sterilization on menstrual indices and pelvic pain. *Obstet Gynecol* **82**(1): 118–21.

Sahwi S, Toppozada M, Kamel M, Anwar MY, Ismail AA (1989) Changes in menstrual blood loss after four methods of female tubal sterilisation. *Contraception* **40**(4): 387–98.

Tang GW, Lo SS (1995) Levonorgestrel intrauterine device in the treatment of menorrhagia in Chinese women: efficacy versus acceptability. *Contraception* **51**(4): 231–5.

Tiltman AJ (1985) The effect of progestins on the mitotic activity of uterine fibromyomas. *Int J Gynecol Pathol* **4**(2): 98–6.

Verco CJ, Carati CJ, Gannon BJ (1998) Human endometrial perfusion after tubal occlusion. *Hum Reprod* **13**(2): 445–9.

Wallach EE (1992) Myomectomy. In: Thompson JD, Rock JA (eds) *Te Linde's Operative Gynecology*, 7th edn, pp 647–62. London: JB Lippincott.

Contraception and amenorrhoea

Nicholas Panay

11

Women who are prescribed certain commonly used hormonal contraceptives will quite often develop amenorrhoea while on these preparations. The issue of whether amenorrhoea develops is dependent on many factors such as the contraceptive method, personal characteristics of the user and ethnic origin (Belsey et al. 1988). The significance of the amenorrhoeic state will be considered in situations where various contraceptives have been prescribed. Through the available published data, this chapter will show how commonly used amenorrhoea-inducing contraceptives may affect, in both the short and long term, the skeletal and cardiovascular system of users. Using this information, practitioners can help their patients make an informed decision as to whether the benefits of continuation of the method outweigh any potential risks that the amenorrhoeic state might bring. The chapter will focus on the consequences of the amenorrhoeic state on the skeletal system in long-term progestogen users, as it is this which has stimulated most controversy and anxiety over the last few years.

Progestogen-only contraception

Long-term continuous progestogens, unopposed by oestrogens, have been in use for contraception for approximately thirty years. Originally, the progestogen-only pill and depot injectables (for example, medroxyprogesterone acetate and hydroxyprogesterone hexanoate) were available. Subdermal levonorgestrel implants were then introduced and have recently been superseded by the removable 3α-ketodesogestrel single rod because of problems with system removal. The levonorgestrel-releasing intrauterine contraceptive device is now available in many countries. All these contraceptives are capable of producing an amenorrhoeic state but with differing significance.

Osteoporosis

During prolonged use of unopposed progestogens, hypothalamic suppression of gonadotrophins can occur, leading to anovulation, with profound decreases in the ovarian production of oestrogen and progesterone and secondary amenorrhoea. This amenorrhoeic state can lead to dramatic changes in bone remodelling with activation of bone-remodelling units, increase in osteoclastic resorption and decrease in bone formation. This leads to rapid loss of trabecular bone, up to 10% in one year (Barengolts et al. 1990). The anxiety which has arisen in the use of long-term progestogens is because, in a significant proportion of people, they lead to this hypooestrogenic, hypoprogestogenic and amenorrhoeic state which could theoretically predispose users to bone loss.

The situation is complicated by the bone trophic effects of progestogens

These effects could potentially compensate for the amenorrhoeic state. We will first consider the data which suggest that progestogens may have a bone-sparing effect. The available data will then be reviewed for the more commonly used amenorrhoea-inducing progestogenic preparations.

Effects of progesterone and progestogens on bone remodelling

In vitro evidence

Discovery of progesterone receptors in human osteoblast-like cells (Erikssen et al. 1988; Komm et al. 1988) provided strong evidence for the mechanism of action of progesterone on bone. In the last few years, progesterone and other progestogens have been shown to directly stimulate osteoblast proliferation in vitro (Tremollieres et al. 1992; Tertinegg and Heersche 1993) suggesting that the effect on bone is in the formation phase of the bone-remodelling cycle.

Animal models

In a study on oophorectomized rats, Lindsay et al. (1978) found that a progestogen, ethynodiol diacetate, prevented loss of bone density from the femur over a 10-month period. Animal study data also indicate that medroxyprogesterone can activate bone remodelling (Karambolova et al. 1986) and increase bone formation in oophorectomized animals and that progesterone can decrease trabecular bone resorption (Barengolts et al. 1990).

Menstrual cycle studies

Prior (1990) postulated a hypothetical relationship between phases of the bone-remodelling cycle and the normal menstrual cycle. Ovarian steroid levels are low at menstruation so increased bone resorption occurs. Increasing oestrogen production before ovulation starts to reverse the resorption. The bone-remodelling units then begin a phase of formation as progesterone levels peak in the midluteal phase. Prior et al. (1990) went on to study 66 premenopausal women over one year. Although nearly all of these women continued to have regular 30-day periods, ovulatory

disturbances such as anovulatory cycles and short luteal phases occurred in 29% of all cycles. These asymptomatic subtle ovulatory disturbances correlated with decreases in spinal bone density. Those women with the most shortened luteal phases (i.e. decreased progesterone production) had the greatest decline in spinal bone density, losing 2–4% of bone per annum.

The maintenance of peak bone density throughout adulthood requires normal ovarian production of progesterone, as well as oestrogen

A subsequent study by Prior et al. (1994a) in women with hypothalamic secondary amenorrhoea, showed that the annual change in spinal bone density was significantly related to the cyclical dose of medroxyprogesterone acetate they received (*Figure 1*). Prior et al. (1994b) then went on to show that cyclical progesterone or other progestogens given as treatment for menstrual cycle disturbances could promote increased bone density. Medroxyprogesterone acetate (10 mg) used for 10 days each month in athletic women with secondary amenorrhoea led to significant

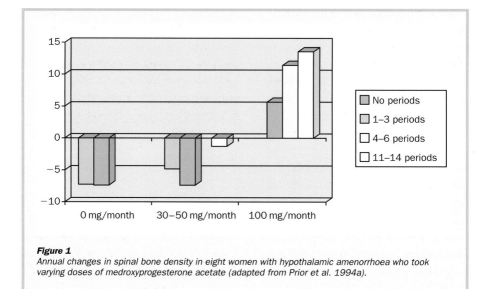

Figure 1
Annual changes in spinal bone density in eight women with hypothalamic amenorrhoea who took varying doses of medroxyprogesterone acetate (adapted from Prior et al. 1994a).

increases in spinal trabecular bone. The inference from all these studies was that continuous progestogens suppress endogenous progesterone levels whereas cyclical progesterone supports the ovarian cycle in the luteal phase and has a bone trophic action.

'Add-back' studies
Add-back therapy studies have been conducted in premenopausal women where gonadotrophin-releasing hormone (GnRH) analogues are given to stop oestrogen production and progestogens are added back to determine whether they have any effect on factors such as hot flushes or bone loss. The

usefulness of these studies in determining the effect on bone of long-term progestogens like depot medroxyprogesterone acetate is that the amenorrhoeic hypoestrogenic state caused by these progestogens can be likened to that produced by gonadotrophin analogues. If the addition of progestogen in these studies does not lead to prevention of bone loss, this suggests that the hypoestrogenic, potentially bone catabolic, state produced by long-term progestogens will not be compensated for by any bone trophic effects of the progestogen itself, leading to osteoporosis. In a study by Riis et al. (1990) the effects of a GnRH analogue, 400 mg nafareline combined with

1.2 mg norethisterone daily for six months were compared to data from a previous six-month study of 400 mg nafarelin alone in women with endometriosis. In the group receiving add-back treatment, the biochemical parameter of bone resorption (fasting urinary hydroxyproline) remained virtually unchanged, compared to a highly significant increase in the nafarelin-alone group. These data were strongly suggestive of a bone-sparing effect for the progestogen. Surrey et al. (1990) used increasing doses of norethisterone (0.35–2.5 mg) in women with endometriosis receiving a GnRH analogue and amongst other outcome measures, the effect on bone mass was evaluated. Bone mineral density of the distal radius was not reduced during therapy but quantitative computed tomography of the lumbar spine after 24 weeks' treatment showed a small but significant decrease in density. Treatment was stopped at 24 weeks and bone density returned to pretreatment levels by 48 weeks. This suggested a bone-sparing effect for cortical but not for vertebral bone; it is possible that if a larger dose had been used, a universal effect would have been seen. Finally, in a prospective, randomised double-blind cross-over study by Breslau et al. (1989), 20 women with endometriosis or fibroids were treated with medroxyprogesterone, 20 mg daily for either the first or second three months and with a GnRH analogue, leuprolide, for six months. The addition of

progestogen led to a decline of fasting and 24-hour calcium levels and hydroxyproline levels suggesting a reduction of bone resorption. Unfortunately, there are no add-back data in any studies on the effect of progestogens on fracture rates which is the most important endpoint for evaluation of agents in osteoporosis treatment.

Osteoporosis and depot medroxyprogesterone acetate (Depo-Provera®)

Concerns about Depo-Provera and osteoporosis first arose from the paper published by Cundy et al. (1991). This cross-sectional study suggested that Depo-Provera, by reducing circulating oestrogen levels, could produce a temporary menopausal state, thus inducing bone atrophy in some users (*Figure 2*). This study was criticized in a number of ways. Firstly, it did not control for other factors such as duration and frequency of smoking, alcohol, parity and other contraceptive methods used. Secondly, and more seriously, there were no pretreatment data. Thirdly, there was inadequate matching of control groups (Hinchley 1991; Szarewski et al. 1991; Kubba 1991). No effect on bone turnover was found by the study; this may be because the treatment led to reduced bone formation rather than increased turnover (Tobias et al. 1991). Reduced formation is more likely to have resulted from reduced oestrogen levels rather than an inhibitory action of

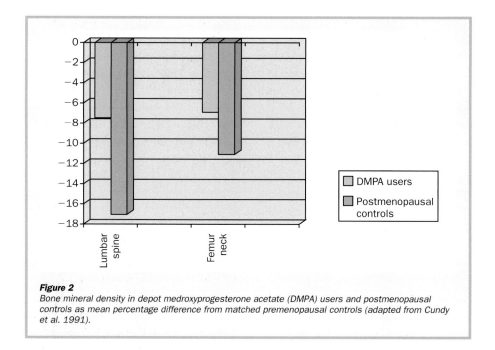

Figure 2
Bone mineral density in depot medroxyprogesterone acetate (DMPA) users and postmenopausal controls as mean percentage difference from matched premenopausal controls (adapted from Cundy et al. 1991).

medroxyprogesterone judging by the trophic effects of the progestogen previously discussed. There was a strong view that a larger prospective randomized controlled study was required to settle the issue.

Cundy et al. (1994) then found that if oestrogen levels returned to normal following cessation of Depo-Provera, spinal bone density returned to almost pretreatment levels. This suggested that the loss of bone density in long-term users was due to the induced

oestrogen deficiency. Changes in the femoral neck were less striking but nonetheless, densities were maintained in women that stopped using Depo-Provera. This study also showed that the women remaining on Depo-Provera from the first study showed no difference in change in bone mass over time from the group which had never used it.

More recent data in adolescent girls (Cromer et al. 1996), also suggest that bone density decreases in Depo-Provera users; a 1.5% decline was detected after one year of usage. However, Kirkman et al. (1994) found maintenance of normal bone density in a small group of women on depot medroxyprogesterone selected by low serum oestradiol and amenorrhoea from their three times greater number of long-term Depo-Provera users without these symptoms. The latest data from this unit and Portsmouth (Gbolade et al. 1998) show that, despite amenorrhoea and low serum oestradiol, this sample of long-term users had bone density only minimally below normal population mean: Z score (age-matched density), lumbar spine -0.332 (95% confidence interval -0.510–0.154).

In view of the questions raised by the Cundy and other data, the manufacturers of Depo-Provera recommend that women who are considered to be at particular risk of osteoporosis whilst on contraception should have their bone density screened and management decided upon those results.

Women entering their normal menopause after prolonged use of Depo-Provera should be strongly considered as candidates for HRT

Using Depo-Provera as the progestogen part of hormone-replacement therapy (HRT) is a very acceptable way of providing continuous combined non-bleed HRT and contraception in the climacteric. Others have suggested the performance of bone densitometry in long-term users with amenorrhoea (Kirkman et al. 1994) and measuring oestradiol levels in long-term users (Szarewski et al. 1994) checking bone densities in those with persistently low levels and adding oestrogens if necessary. However, oestradiol assays can be unreliable at low levels and what may be normal for one person may be pathological for another. Therefore, if there is any doubt about the oestradiol levels, bone densitometry should be performed.

A position paper has recently been produced on the clinical use and side effects of Depo-Provera (Bigrigg et al. 1999). The group state that the menstrual disturbances caused by Depo-Provera can be improved by giving short courses of oestrogen.

Add-back therapy should minimize the risk of osteoporosis

The risk is minimized due to the hypo-oestrogenic state induced by long-term usage. Menstrual irregularity and risk of bone loss can be avoided by the use of the newly developed

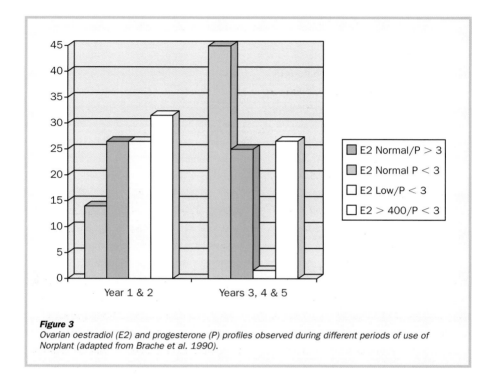

Figure 3
Ovarian oestradiol (E2) and progesterone (P) profiles observed during different periods of use of Norplant (adapted from Brache et al. 1990).

combined monthly injectable contraceptives. Two preparations, Cyclofem and Mesigyna, already available in some countries, still provide the convenience and contraceptive efficacy of depot injections in women who do not have a contraindication to oestrogen (Newton 1996). The general consensus is that until the case for Depo-Provera and osteoporosis is proven, it should continue to be widely used as it not only provides excellent contraceptive protection but also gives a fivefold protective effect against endometrial cancer (Szarewski et al. 1994). It is strongly felt in the position paper that as Depo-Provera is a highly effective contraceptive with few risks, that 'it should be available as a first line method to all who wish to make an informed choice about reversible methods of contraception'.

Osteoporosis and progestogen implants (Norplant®/Implanon®)

In order to assess the risk of osteoporosis in women using progestogen implants, we must extrapolate from studies of serum oestradiol levels as few bone-density and no fracture data are available. Alvarez et al. (1986) measured hormone levels in eight cycles in six Norplant (subdermal implants: 6 rods containing 228 mg of levonorgestrel) acceptors for a period of two to four years. No significant differences were observed in oestradiol levels between Norplant users and controls. In a longer-term study, Croxatto et al. (1988) studied 47 women using Norplant for seven years. In only one woman were her oestradiol levels consistently below 370 pmol/l. Brache et al. (1990) studied 92 cycles (*Figure 3*). In approximately one out of every four cycles during the first two years of Norplant use and one in twenty cycles in the third year of use, low oestradiol levels were found. With use after the third year however, no low oestradiol levels were observed. However, the sampling method used in this study i.e. 10 samples taken in a five-week period, may have been adequate to determine the proportion of cycles with luteal activity but not necessarily to define persistently low oestrogen secretion. In only three of the 92 observed cycles were oestrogen levels maintained below 147 pmol/l during sampling and this was in women with weight below 55 kg.

Women with low body weight are at greater risk of ovarian suppression due to higher levonorgestrel levels and hence at risk of osteoporosis

A much longer study would be required to determine how long these low oestradiol levels are maintained.

Implanon, has recently been licensed as a single removable rod containing the third-generation 19-nortestosterone-derived 3-ketodesogestrel applied subdermally. In a recent study by Croxatto et al. (1998), ovulation inhibition was determined by serum progesterone levels and ultrasound scanning of the ovaries. Ovarian function was further assessed by serum oestradiol levels. Inhibition of ovulation, reflected by suppressed progesterone levels, was the primary mode of action. Although ovulation was inhibited, ovarian activity was still present judging by follicle growth and oestradiol synthesis. The follicle-stimulating hormone (FSH) serum concentrations were only slightly lower than pre-insertion levels and leuteinizing hormone (LH) surges were prevented. Return of ovulation after removal of Implanon was rapid. In a further multicentre study (Croxatto et al. 1999) involving 635 young healthy women, although bleeding irregularities were the main reason for discontinuation during the first two years of use (17.2%), return of fertility was prompt owing to preservation of follicular activity. The safety profile was acceptable and not dissimilar to progestogens in general. With Implanon there is preservation of follicular activity with normal FSH and oestradiol levels

There should be no significant risk of osteoporosis with Implanon

Progesterone levels during use of Norplant and Implanon are significantly lower as compared with controls. Assuming a bone trophic action for progesterone, as discussed earlier, this might predispose to osteoporosis.

Norplant increases bone density in adolescent girls

Bone density is increased by 2.5% after one year and 9.3% after two years, probably due to the maintenance of follicular activity and an additive bone trophic effect (Cromer et al. 1996). It could be extrapolated from this that Implanon would have the same effect though bone-density studies are required to confirm this.

Osteoporosis and the progestogen-only pill (POP)

It is known that approximately 16% of women using the progestogen-only pill are amenorrhoeic, with diminished follicular activity, low oestrogen levels, no corpus luteum formation and no endogenous progesterone production (Guillebaud 1997). This situation is ideal from the point of view of contraception, but well may predispose them to increased bone turnover and ultimately osteoporosis. In view of the very small doses of progestogen used in the POP the 'add-back' effect in these women will be minimal, thus compounding the problem.

In the absence of any good data on this issue, Guillebaud (1997) recommends that after five years' POP amenorrhoea, women, especially smokers, should have plasma oestradiol checked and a bone-density scan performed. If the oestradiol levels are less than 100 pmol/l or the scan shows osteoporosis, it is recommended that either another contraceptive method should be chosen or consideration should be given to adding-back natural oestrogen by any chosen route. Guillebaud adds that even if the tests are not available, the POP should be continued unless the woman has symptoms of oestrogen deficiency.

Women with long-term amenorrhoea should not be banned from using the POP

It is clear that a long-term prospective study is required so that clear guidelines can be given to women using this form of contraception, particularly if they are amenorrhoeic.

Levonorgestrel intrauterine system (Mirena®)

The 20 µg over 24 hours levonorgestrel-releasing intrauterine contraceptive device is now licensed to provide contraception for five years after insertion. Approximately 20% of women will become amenorrhoeic after one year; this may raise some anxiety as to predisposition to osteoporosis with long-term usage. Also, because systemic absorption is so little, the add-back effect would be minimal. However, oligomenorrhoea is produced by local prevention of endometrial proliferation. Despite prevention of ovulation in some cycles (Nilsson et al. 1984) work has been done to show that plasma oestradiol levels remain within the normal range for fertile women (Luukkainen et al. 1990), so there should be no predisposition to osteoporosis. Ideally, the prospective studies should have studied bone densities and markers of bone turnover for the definitive answer.

Cardiovascular disease

There does not appear to be an increase in cardiovascular mortality or morbidity in amenorrhoeic users of long-term progestogenic contraception. However, the reports on long-term progestogens and markers for cardiovascular disease are inconsistent, probably due to variable methodology. Changes in metabolic cardiovascular markers are dependent on the steroid content and dosage and the method of delivery. Also, there are very few data on the effect that amenorrhoea specifically has on the cardiovascular risk markers. One might postulate that in hypoestrogenic amenorrhoeic users, there would be absence of beneficial opposition to the adverse effects that most progestogens have on cardiovascular risk factors. In making decisions for our patients we can only take the data as a whole and extrapolate from this. The specific risk for each amenorrhoeic individual will be dependent on personal and family history of cardiovascular disease, smoking, obesity, hypertension, as well as duration of hypoestrogenic state. The existing data for cardiovascular risk of all users (including amenorrhoeic patients) of long-term progestogens will now be considered to determine what the risk may be for the amenorrhoeic subset.

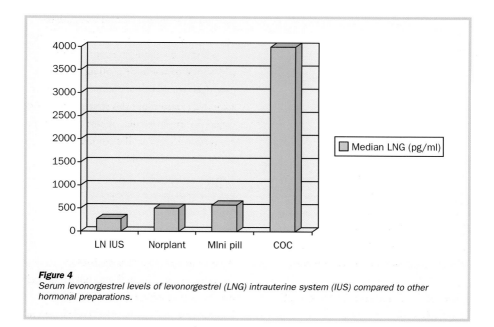

Figure 4
Serum levonorgestrel levels of levonorgestrel (LNG) intrauterine system (IUS) compared to other hormonal preparations.

In long-term progestogen users as a whole, changes in lipids/lipoproteins remain within the normal range, suggesting that there would be no significant effect on the rate of development of cardiovascular disease. The changes which do occur in cardiovascular markers are inconsistent. There is a beneficial lowering of total triglyceride and cholesterol levels but a detrimental increase in low-density lipoprotein (LDL) levels reported in some studies (Johansson and Odlind 1983). Other studies suggest a deleterious effect on high-density lipoprotein (HDL) levels with a 15–20% reduction quoted in some studies (Deslypere et al. 1985; Fahmy et al. 1991). Even with the low levels of progestogen released by the levonorgestrel intrauterine system (*Figure 4*), some women still seem to experience adverse metabolic effects with decreased HDL levels (Raudaskoski et al. 1995). However, it is uncertain whether lowering of absolute serum HDL levels increases the risk of cardiovascular disease as there may be a normal transportation of cholesterol from the vessel wall to the liver despite reduced HDL (Crook 1999, personal communication).

None of the progestogen-only long-acting methods appear to have clinically significant effects on carbohydrate metabolism

This is despite an impairment of the oral glucose tolerance test by Depo-Provera of the same order as the oral contraceptive pill. (Weisberg and Fraser 1998). However, no previously normal subject has developed diabetes as a result of these treatments.

With regards to the other risk factors of coagulation and blood pressure, yet again, there appears to be no significant effect whether the patient is amenorrhoeic or not. In a study by McEwan and Griffin (1991) the majority of users of depot norethisterone enanthate had experienced amenorrhoea for more than two consecutive injection intervals. There was no significant difference in factor VIIIc, Xc, antithrombin III or haemoglobin levels over controls.

In summary, the overall data show no significant risk of cardiovascular disease with long-term progestogenic users. However, in those amenorrhoeic users who are hypo-oestrogenic and have significant personal or family history it is advisable to perform

lipid/lipoprotein/oral glucose tolerance test estimation (where available). If adverse trends are detected, an alternative contraceptive or addition of oestradiol (e.g. 50 µg oestradiol patch/gel) would be the options. It would be advisable to also adopt this strategy where risk factors for cardiovascular disease exist in hypo-oestrogenic users even if cardiovascular markers are not available.

Combined oral contraceptive (COC)

Osteoporosis

Women using the COC who develop amenorrhoea may do so during pill use or find they have 'post-pill amenorrhoea'. The amenorrhoea during pill usage is of concern to the user because they may start to question whether they have fallen pregnant. Assuming all pills have been taken and there has not been a reason for malabsorption, e.g. gastroenteritis, these women can be reassured that there is no medical reason to discontinue or change the preparation. The oestrogen in the pill will protect the skeleton and lack of bleeding is not a sign of a hypo-oestrogenic state (albeit that the oestrogen is exogenous). Should the user be unhappy with the amenorrhoeic state they can be switched to a more oestrogen-dominant pill which should restore withdrawal bleeds. The amenorrhoea is probably a combination of progestogen dominance and sensitive progestogen receptors in the endometrium.

It is widely accepted that post-pill amenorrhoea is not as a result of the pill but that amenorrhoea was merely masked by the withdrawal bleeds induced by the pill. This is supported by evidence showing that the incidence of amenorrhoea in young women is exactly the same whether they have used the COC or not. The causes of such amenorrhoea fall into four broad categories:

- Hypothalamic, e.g. weight loss/exercise related: These women are usually hypo-oestrogenic and require referral for baseline bone densitometry and ongoing therapy with preferably non-oral oestrogens and progestogens (although the pill can be continued).

- Polycystic ovarian syndrome: Women with PCOS are usually normally or hyper-oestrogenized. They therefore do not require bone-density monitoring or supplemental oestrogen though they should have cyclical progestogen or continue the COC in order to protect the endometrium from hyperplasia.

- Hyperprolactinaemia: A referral to an endocrinologist for an MRI of the pituitary fossa and probable treatment with bromocriptine is indicated. Oestradiol levels should be monitored.

- Amenorrhoea with normal oestrogenization: Here there is evidence of some follicular activity but no ovulation. Reassurance is usually all that is required and there is no reason why the pill could not be continued in order to provide some endometrial protection.

Combined oral contraceptive use increases bone mass

The data that COC use increases bone mass do not refer to amenorrhoeic patients specifically. However, the absence of withdrawal bleeds is usually a sign of progestogen dominance; oestrogenization is similar whether there is bleeding or not. The general data should therefore be representative of the amenorrhoeic subset. Cromer et al. (1996) showed in their prospective study that those adolescent girls receiving the oral contraceptive pill had an increase in bone mineral density of 1.5% after one year. A cross-sectional retrospective study found that those women who had been oral contraceptive users in the past had significantly higher bone mineral density than those who had not used oral contraceptives. The longer the duration of use, the higher bone density was found to be (Kleerkoper et al. 1991). In a 36-month prospective study of perimenopausal women, there was preservation of bone mass in the

Table 1
Possibility of skeletal/cardiovascular risk with different amenorrhoea-inducing contraceptive preparations.

Preparation	Risk of osteoporosis	Risk of cardiovascular disease
Depo-Provera	Some data suggesting possible risk but prospective randomized controlled trial data needed	Possible risk from reduced HDL and increased insulin resistance but no increased incidence of myocardial infarction
Norplant/Implanon	Limited but reassuring data	Possible risk to lipids/lipoproteins – no increased incidence of myocardial infarction
Progestogen-only pill	No data – randomized controlled trial data needed	Possible risk to lipids/lipoproteins – no increased incidence of myocardial infarction
Mirena	No evidence of any risk	Possible risk to lipids/lipoproteins – no increased incidence of myocardial infarction
Combined oral contraceptive	Evidence of beneficial effect	No evidence of increased myocardial infarction risk

100 women who received a triphasic oral contraceptive whereas the 100 controls lost approximately 6% of their bone mass (Shargil 1985).

Cardiovascular disease

To determine the risk to the cardiovascular system, once again we can look at surrogate markers for cardiovascular disease. Oral oestrogens increase the level of HDLs and decrease the level of LDLs. These changes are thought to be favourable from the point of view of cardiovascular disease. Progestogens have the opposite effect depending on how androgenic they are in their effect. The net effect of a particular COC depends on the dominance of oestrogen versus progestogen and the type of progestogen used. In preparations containing levonorgestrel, there may be a significant reduction in HDL levels (Godsland et al. 1990). In principle, it is better to use a contraceptive which has the least adverse effect on metabolic risk factors

Table 2
Summary of management of long-term amenorrhoea induced by different contraceptive preparations.

Preparation	Management guidelines (long term amenorrhoea)
Depo-Provera	Monitor oestradiol levels ± bone mineral density Use combined injectable (where available) or add-back natural oestrogen or . . . Switch to other method such as Implanon
Norplant/Implanon	Monitor with oestradiol levels Bone mineral density and cardiovascular markers if oestradiol persistently low (unlikely) Switch method/add-back oestradiol if risk factors
Progestogen-only pill	Exclude pregnancy Monitor oestradiol levels if amenorrhoea over five years or if risk factors for osteoporosis/cardiovascular disease Bone mineral density if oestradiol persistently low Discontinue or add-back oestradiol, if low oestradiol + low bone mineral density
Mirena	Reassure patient that amenorrhoea is due to mechanism of action Lipids/lipoproteins if risk factors for cardiovascular disease
Combined oral contraceptive	Exclude pregnancy if missed pills/reasons for malabsorption Reassure patient that no risk If patient worried about amenorrhoea, switch to more oestrogen-dominant pill

Exclude pregnancy for Mirena/Norplant/Depo-Provera only if patient anxious or if clinical indication to do so, e.g. late with depot injections/expelled Mirena.

(Fotherby 1990). Recent studies have shown no increase in risk of myocardial infarction either during or after COC usage (Thorneycroft 1990, Rosenberg et al. 1990, Thorogood et al. 1991; Colditz 1994). It would be expected that these findings were independent of menstrual state during COC usage.

It is the synthetic not endogenous oestrogen, which provides the favourable effect on the markers for cardiovascular disease

Cigarette smoking by oral contraceptive users is the predominant associated risk factor for the occurrence of arterial disease (Kay 1984).

As far as post-pill amenorrhoea is concerned, the risk for myocardial infarction will be dependent on the aetiology. In normally oestrogenized women, there should be no excess risk. However, women with polycystic ovarian syndrome are thought to have insulin resistance and this is an additional risk factor for future myocardial infarction. Hypo-oestrogenic women should be given oestrogen supplementation in order to reduce the risk of an adverse on lipids/lipoproteins/insulin resistance.

Conclusions (*Tables 1 and 2*)

Review of the data available for progestogenic contraceptives such as depot medroxyprogesterone acetate and the progestogen-only pill provide inconclusive evidence as to the magnitude of risk for loss of bone density in amenorrhoeic users. Although these progestogens continue to be bone trophic in long-term usage, this may not fully compensate the increased bone turnover and resorption due to the hypo-oestrogenic amenorrhoea which they can cause. Large long-term randomized controlled studies are required, examining biochemical bone markers, densities and fracture data to resolve the issue. Until those studies are done we must continue to be vigilant, particularly when using long-term unopposed progestogen. If in any doubt, it would seem sensible to have a low threshold for performing oestradiol levels, serial bone densitometry and markers where available. Levonorgestrel/etonogestrel implants and the levonorgestrel intrauterine system should not predispose users to bone loss as follicular activity and in the case of the latter, ovulation, are maintained. The combined oral contraceptives contain ethinyloestradiol which protects the skeleton whether there is amenorrhoea or not. As far as cardiovascular risk is concerned, there is a paucity of data from which to determine the specific risk of amenorrhoea in users of these contraceptive methods. In general, there is no increased risk of myocardial infarction with long-term use of any of these methods and factors such as smoking and obesity are more important than an amenorrhoeic state. However, with contraceptive preparations where amenorrhoeic users are often hypo-oestrogenic, such as with Depo-Provera, it would seem prudent to advise a switch to an alternative contraceptive method in women with cardiovascular risk factors such as a significant personal/family history or poor lipid/lipoprotein/insulin resistance profile. The practice of giving add-back oestrogen should also be encouraged as this provides a good option for the amenorrhoeic hypo-oestrogenic progestogen user who does not have contraindications. On present evidence, there is little doubt that, even for amenorrhoeic users, the benefits of all the contraceptive methods discussed in this chapter far outweigh their risks.

Case histories

Case 1

Margaret, a 45-year-old caucasian woman, had been using Depo-Provera since completing her family of two children 10 years ago. She had been completely amenorrhoeic for the last five years and her family doctor was concerned about the publicity regarding long-term progestogens and the possible risks of osteoporosis, particularly in women who do not menstruate. In view of this concern, she was referred to a gynaecological endocrinologist for assessment and further management.

'I'm happy not to have periods and want to carry on with the injections, but I'm worried now,' she says. There was no significant personal or family history of osteoporosis-related factors. However, a hypo-oestrogenic state was detected with a serum oestradiol of 72 pmol/l. Bone density was slightly below the age-matched bone density of 90% (Z score -0.5).

The advice given was that either the Depo-Provera could be stopped and an alternative method chosen or the depot could be continued but with oestradiol add-back therapy given, such as a 50 µg oestradiol patch changed twice weekly. She decided to continue with the Depo-Provera plus add-back therapy. Monitoring of oestradiol levels was performed on a six-monthly basis and bone densitometry was carried out on an annual basis. As she advanced into the peri-menopausal years, this regimen not only proved to be a good contraceptive but also fulfilled the needs of hormone replacement therapy.

Case 2

Adrienne, a 30-year-old multiparous woman, smoked 20 cigarettes per day and had been using the combined oral contraceptive, microgynon, for contraception for 5 years. She visited her family doctor for a routine check-up. She was generally happy with the contraceptive but had not had a withdrawal bleed for the last 12 months. Of significance, her mother, now in her 60s, had recently suffered a myocardial infarction. Her doctor was concerned that this amenorrhoeic state might predispose her patient to osteoporosis and the risk of cardiovascular disease in the long-term, particularly in view of her smoking habits. She referred Adrienne to the family planning clinic for further assessment.

'My mum didn't take the pill, so I'm sure it's not the problem,' she says. A general examination revealed no abnormalities. A hormone profile revealed a low oestradiol level, and a thrombophilia screen and lipid profile proved to be normal apart from a reduced high-density lipoprotein (HDL) level.

Adrienne was reassured that there should be no increased risk of osteoporosis from the amenorrhoeic state. Although ovulation was suppressed, the ethinyloestradiol should more than adequately counterbalance this endogenous hypo-oestrogenic state to prevent any increased risk of osteoporosis, However, she was advised that smoking would increase her risk of both osteoporosis and cardiovascular disease; particularly in view of her family history, it would be wise to try to reduce or – better still – stop smoking. In view of the reduced HDL levels and family history of cardiovascular disease, she was switched to a pill with a less androgenic progestogen (desogestrel). She was warned that her bleeds might well recommence on this pill in view of the less androgenic progestogen.

References

Alvarez F, Brache V, Tedaja AS et al. (1986) Abnormal endocrine profile among women with confirmed or presumed ovulation during long term Norplant use. *Contraception* 33: 111–19.

Barengolts EI, Gajardo HF, Rusol TJ et al. (1990) Effects of progesterone and postovariectomy bone loss in aged rats. *J Bone Min Res* 5: 1143–7.

Belsey EM, Peregoudov S and Task Force on Long Acting Systemic Agents for Fertility Regulation (1988) Determinants of menstrual bleeding patterns among women using natural and hormonal methods of contraception. *Contraception* 32(2): 227–35.

Bigrigg A, Evans M, Gbolade B et al. (1999) Depo-Provera Position paper on clinical use, effectiveness and side effects. *Br J Fam Plann* **25**: 69–76.

Brache V, Alvarez-Sanchez F, Faundes A et al. (1990) Ovarian endocrine function through five years of continuous treatment with Norplant subdermal contraceptive implants. *Contraception* **41**: 169–75.

Breslau NA, Steinkampf MP, Bradshaw KD et al. (1989) Amelioration of GnRH-induced calcium loss by progesterone (Abstract 482). *J Bone Min Res* **4**: S238.

Colditz GA (1994) The Nurse's Health Study Research Group. Oral contraceptive use and mortality during 12 years of follow-up: the Nurse's Health Study. *Ann Int Med* **120**: 821–6.

Cromer BA, Blair JM, Mahan JD (1996) A prospective comparison of bone density in adolescent girls receiving depot medroxyprogesterone acetate (Depo-Provera), levonorgestrel (Norplant), or oral contraceptives. *J Padiatr* **129**: 671–6.

Croxatto HB, Makarainen L (1998) The pharmacodynamics and efficacy of Implanon. An overview of the data. *Contraception* **58**(6 Suppl): 91S–97S.

Croxatto HB, Soledad D, Pavez M et al. (1988) Oestradiol plasma levels during long term treatment with Norplant subdermal implants. *Contraception* **38**(4): 465–74.

Croxatto HB, Urbancsek J, Massai R et al. (1999) A multicentre efficacy and safety study of the single contraceptive implant Implanon. Implanon Study Group. *Hum Reprod* **14**(4): 976–81.

Cundy T, Evans E, Roberts H et al. (1991) Bone density in women receiving depot medroxyprogesterone acetate for contraception. *Br Med J* **303**: 13–16.

Cundy T, Cornish J, Evans MC et al. (1994) Recovery of bone density in women who stopped using medroxyprogesterone acetate. *Br Med J* **308**: 247–8.

Deslypere JF, Thiery M, Vermeulen A (1985) Effect of long-term hormonal contraception on plasma lipids. *Contraception* **31**: 633–42.

Erikssen EF, Colvard DS, Berg NJ et al. (1988) Evidence of oestrogen receptors in normal human osteoblast-like cells. *Science* **241**: 84.

Fahmy K, Khairy M, Allam G (1991) Effect of depo-medroxyprogesterone acetate on coagulation factors and serum lipids in Egyptian women. *Contraception* **44**: 431–44.

Fotherby K (1990) Update on lipid metabolism and oral contraception. *Br J Fam Plann* **15**: 23–6.

Gbolade B, Ellis S, Murby B et al. (1998) Bone density in long term users of depot medroxyprogesterone acetate. *Br J Obstet Gynaecol* **105**(7): 790–4.

Godsland IF, Crook D, Simpson R et al. (1990) The effects of different formulations of oral contraceptive agents on lipid and carbohydrate metabolism. *New Engl J Med* **323**: 1375–81.

Guillebaud J (1997) Oestrogen-free hormonal contraception. In: *Contraception: Your Questions Answered*, 2nd edn. Edinburgh: Churchill Livingstone.

Hinchley H (1991) DMPA and bone density. *Br Med J* **303**: 467.

Johansson E, Odlind V Norplant: biochemical effects. Long acting steroid contraception. In: Mishell D, ed. *Advance in Human Fertility and Reproductive Endocrinology*, Vol 2. New York: Raven Press, 1983: 117–25.

Karambolova KK, Snow GR, Anderson C (1986) Surface activity on the periosteal and corticoendosteal envelopes following continuous progestogen supplementation in spayed beagles. *Calc Tissue Int* **38**: 239–43.

Kay CR (1984) The Royal College of General Practitioners' Oral Contraception Study: some recent observations. *Clin Obstet Gynaecol* **11**(3): 759–86.

Kirkman R, Williams E, Murby B (1994) Bone

density and use of depot medroxyprogesterone acetate DMPA (Depo-Provera). *Br J Fam Plann* **20**(1): 26–7.

Kleerkoper M, Brienza RS, Schultz LR et al. (1991) Oral contraceptive use may protect against low bone mass: Henry Ford Hospital Osteoporosis Cooperative Research Group. *Arch Int Med* **151**: 1971.

Komm BS, Terpening CM, Benz DJ et al. (1988) Estrogen binding, receptor mRNA and biologic response in osteoblast-like sarcoma cells. *Science* **241**: 81.

Kubba A (1991) DMPA and bone density. *Br Med J* **301**: 467.

Lindsay R, Hart DM, Aitken JM et al. (1978) The effect of ovarian sex steroids on bone mineral status in the oophorectomised rat and in the human. *Postgrad Med* 54S: 50.

Luukkainen T, Lahteenmaki P, Toivonen J (1990) Levonorgestrel-releasing intrauterine device. *Ann Med* **22**(2): 85–90.

McEwan JA, Griffin M (1991) Long-term use of depot-norethisterone enanthate: effect on blood coagulation factors and menstrual bleeding patterns. *Contraception* **44**(6): 639–48.

Newton J (1996) New hormonal methods of contraception. *Baillière's Clin Obstet Gynaecol* **10**(1): 87–101.

Nilsson CG, Lahteenmaki P, Luukkainen T (1984) Ovarian function in amenorrhoeic and menstruating users of a levonorgestrel releasing intrauterine device. *Fertil Steril* **41**: 52–5.

Prior JC (1990) Progesterone as a bone-trophic hormone. *Endocr Rev* **11**: 386–9.

Prior JC, Vigna Y, Schecter MT et al. (1990) Spinal bone loss and ovulatory disturbances. *N Engl J Med* **323**: 1221–7.

Prior JC, Vigna YM, Kennedy SM (1994a) Progesterone's role in bone remodelling. *Br J Fam Plann* **19**(S): 13–17.

Prior JC, Vigna YM, Barr SI et al. (1994b) Cyclic medroxyprogesterone treatment increases

bone density: a controlled trial in active women with menstrual cycle disturbances. *Am J Med* **96**: 521–30.

Raudaskoski TH, Tomas EI, Paakkari IA et al. (1995) Serum lipids and lipoproteins in postmenopausal women receiving transdermal oestrogen in combination with a levonorgestrel intrauterine device. *Maturitas* **22**(1): 47–53.

Riis BJ, Christiansen JS, Johansen JS et al. (1990) Is it possible to prevent bone loss in young women treated with luteinizing hormone-releasing hormone agonists? *J Clin Endocrinol Metab* **70**: 920–4.

Rosenberg L, Palmer JR, Lesko SM, Shapiro S (1990) Oral contraception use and the risk of myocardial infarction. *Am J Epidemiol* **131**: 1009–16.

Shargil AA (1985) Hormone replacement therapy in perimenopausal women with a triphasic contraceptive compound. A three year prospective study. *Intl J Fertil* **30**: 15.

Sivin I (1988) International experience with Norplant and Norplant-2 contraceptives. *Studies Fam Plann* **19**: 81–94.

Surrey ES, Gambone JC, Lu JKH et al. (1990) The effects of combining norethindrone with a gonadotrophin-releasing hormone agonist in the treatment of symptomatic endometriosis. *Fertil Steril* **53**: 620–6.

Szarewski A, Guillebaud J, Christopher E (1991) DMPA and bone density. *Br Med J* **303**: 467.

Szarewski A, Hollingsworth B, Guillebaud J (1994) Depot medroxyprogesterone acetate and osteoporosis. *Br Med J* **308**: 717.

Tertinegg L, Heersche JN (1993) Progesterone stimulates bone nodule formation in rat cadavarial cell cultures while oestrogen has no effect. *J Bone Min Res* **7**: 5220.

Thorneycroft IH (1990) Oral contraceptives and myocardial infarction. *Am J Obstet Gynecol* **163**: 1393–7.

Thorogood M, Mann J, Murphy M, et al. (1991) Is oral contraceptive use still associated with an increased risk of fatal myocardial infarction? Report of a case-controlled study. *Br J Obstet Gynaecol* **98**: 1245–53.

Tobias JH, Chow J, Chambers TJ (1991) DMPA and bone density. *Br Med J* **303**: 468.

Tremollieres FA, Strong DD, Baylink DT et al. (1992) Progesterone and promogesterone stimulate human bone cell proliferation and insulin-like growth factor 2 production. *Acta Endocrinol* **126**: 329–37.

Weisberg E, Fraser I (1998) Clinical aspects of the use of long-acting hormonal contraception. In: Fraser I, Jansen RPS, Lobo RA, Whitehead MI eds. *Estrogens and Progestogens in Clinical Practice*. London: Churchill Livingstone.

WHO Collaborative Study of Neoplasia and Steroid Contraceptives (1991) Depot medroxyprogesterone acetate (DMPA) and risk of endometrial cancer. *Intl J Cancer* **49**: 186–90.

Couples with fertility problems

Stephen Killick

12

There are many instances when those of us who provide advice for couples requiring contraception need to have a working knowledge of subfertility and the way it is commonly managed. Sadly, contraceptive services and fertility services are usually provided by different practitioners and in separate clinical locations. In vitro fertilization (IVF) units tend to be isolated from mainstream medical services for a number of reasons, including funding arrangements, rapidly advancing technology, and the complexities of the confidentiality clause of the Human Fertilisation and Embryology Act.

Contraceptive advice for couples who have a fertility problem would, on the face of it, appear to be nonsense. There are many situations, however, when couples with lower than average fertility will wish to be sure that pregnancy does not occur. In these not uncommon cases contraceptive advice can be difficult and needs to be approached from a slightly different viewpoint to advice given in other circumstances.

Previous contraceptive use is often quoted by subfertile couples as the reason for their problem. This is rarely the case, however, as contraceptive use generally preserves fertility.

Natural fertility

A couple with no barriers to conception cannot expect more than a 1 in 3 chance of pregnancy in any given month of trying. The human species is inferior to others in this respect. Animals such as the rabbit are reflex ovulators and ovulate in response to coitus. Humans are facultative ovulators, trusting that intercourse will probably occur at about the time that an oocyte is released. This does not mean, however, that conception can only occur if coitus takes place at exactly mid-cycle. *Figure 1* shows the probability of conception following a single act of coitus on various days of the menstrual cycle for couples who do not have a fertility problem.

No couple has a greater than 1 in 3 chance of conception per month

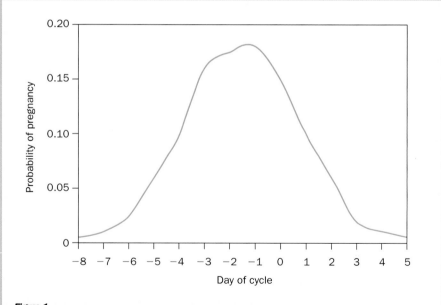

Figure 1
Probability of pregnancy resulting from coitus on a given day of the ovarian cycle in couples with normal fertility. Day 0 represents the day of ovulation.

The probability of conception is an important concept and is a recurring theme throughout this chapter. If all couples had the optimal 1 in 3 chance of conceiving in every cycle then less than 1% would have been unlucky enough not to have done so after 12 months of trying. This is not the case, however, when real populations are studied because some couples are less fertile than others, and 10–15% of couples are found not to have conceived at the end of 1 year. *Figure 2* shows a typical cumulative conception rate curve. Similar curves have been drawn from population studies from all parts of the world. The success rates for repeated attempts at every type of fertility treatment (*Figure 3*) and the failure rates of all forms of contraception (*Figure 4*) also follow this curve. It is therefore fundamental to the understanding of fertility.

Subfertility is usually defined as the inability to conceive after 1 year of regular coitus, but because this definition results in such a high prevalence (more than 10% of the entire population), some authorities prefer a definitive period of 2 years of regular coitus.

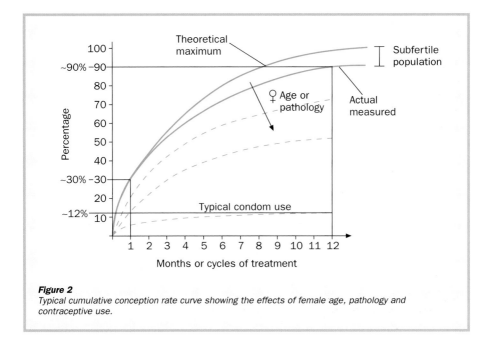

Figure 2
Typical cumulative conception rate curve showing the effects of female age, pathology and contraceptive use.

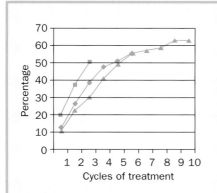

Figure 3
Cumulative pregnancy rates from repeated
cycles of IVF treatment. Data from Guzick et
al. (1986) (diamonds), de Mouzon et
al. (1988) (squares) and Dor et al. (1996)
(triangles). Note the similarity to the curves in
Figure 2. The actual numerical values should
not be compared as the rates were
calculated using different methods.

The term 'subfertility' is preferred to
'infertility' because although fertility rates can
become extremely low it is unwise ever to
pronounce a couple to be absolutely sterile.
All sterilization procedures have a failure rate
(about 4% over 10 years) and there have even
been recorded cases of live delivery by
laparotomy after hysterectomy and despite
congenital vaginal atresia.

Many factors will lower the cumulative
pregnancy rate curve, including smoking,
coital frequency and various pathological
disorders of both the male and female partner.

The most important factor is female age.
Women are born with all the oocytes they will
ever have, each one destined to develop in
preparation for ovulation at a predetermined
time. It appears that oocytes that are released
earlier in life are of a higher quality than those
that are released later. Older oocytes have less
chance of fertilization. Furthermore, even if
they are fertilized they have less chance of
implantation; if they implant they have a
higher chance of miscarriage; and if they do
not miscarry they have a higher chance of
chromosomal abnormality. Natural
conception rates begin to fall slowly at the age
of 30 years. Therefore, the best we can hope
for with any form of fertility treatment is a
success rate equivalent to natural cumulative
pregnancy rates for women of the same age.
An exception to this is when a woman is
treated with donated oocytes from a younger
woman, when not only are her chances of
pregnancy greater than would be expected for
her age but also her chances of miscarriage or
of a chromosomally abnormal child are much
reduced.

*Fertility begins to fall
after the age of 30 years
in women*

Contraception can be viewed in exactly the
same way, although the cumulative pregnancy

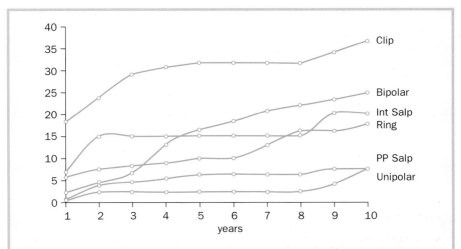

Figure 4
Failure rates of sterilization after different surgical procedures according to the US collaborative survey of 1996. The vertical scale is per 1000 procedures per year. Failure rates all decrease with time; this is not so pronounced for diathermy techniques, probably because of the risk of tubal recannulation. Key to methods: Clip, tubal clip; Bipolar, bipolar diathermy; Int Salp, interval salpingectomy; Ring, Fallope ring; PP Salp, post-partum salpingectimy, Unipolar, unipolar diathermy. Data from Peterson et al (1996).

rate is much lower and is viewed as failure rather than success. Failure rates of virtually all contraceptive methods diminish with increasing duration of use.

Contraception and future fertility

Couples often relate a fertility problem to their past contraceptive use even though contraception generally serves to preserve fertility.

Contraception generally serves to preserve fertility

Post-pill amenorrhoea

The most obvious example of this phenomenon is post-pill amenorrhoea. A woman will report that she experienced regular periods before she started combined oral contraception and also regular withdrawal bleeds while she took it, but that her periods failed to return once she stopped therapy. To her mind the pill must have caused the problem.

In the majority of these cases, however, the cause of the amenorrhoea dates from a change at some time during the pill-taking years which was masked by pill use. Hence the longer the duration of pill use, the more likely the chance of amenorrhoea. Common examples of causes, in decreasing order of frequency, are polycystic ovary syndrome, weight-related amenorrhoea, and hyperprolactinaemia. These patients should have their basal metabolic index recorded and blood taken for assessment of follicle-stimulating hormone, luteinizing hormone and prolactin. Thyrotoxicosis is also relatively common in young women but rarely presents with amenorrhoea as the only symptom.

The incidence of post-pill amenorrhoea lasting for 6 months or more is about 1 in 200 and about half of these cases resolve spontaneously before 1 year (Jones 1977). Factors said to increase the likelihood of post-pill amenorrhoea are, not surprisingly, a late menarche, previous oligomenorrhoea and low body weight (Weisberg 1982). Appropriate treatment results in pregnancy rates of over 90% within 1 year (Hull et al. 1981).

In a proportion of individuals the amenorrhoea appears to be a true post-pill phenomenon. In these cases a short course of clomiphene citrate is usually enough to reinstate a normal menstrual cycle. This is usually given after a negative pregnancy test in doses of 50 mg or 100 mg daily for 5 days. Women who develop true post-pill amenorrhoea tend to be those who respond to other stimuli throughout their lives with periods of oligomenorrhoea or amenorrhoea.

Post-pill amenorrhoea is usually caused by the same factors that lead to amenorrhoea in other situations

Delayed fertility following use of depot progestogens

Medroxyprogesterone acetate (MPA) is detected in the serum as quickly as 30 minutes after an intramuscular injection of 150 mg of the depot preparation. Levels remain constant at about 1.0 ng/ml for 3 months and then steadily decrease over the next 6 months (Mishell 1996), during which time fertility gradually returns; the mean time to conception has been recorded as 9.2 months (Fraser and Dennerstein 1994). The delay in fertility may occasionally be as long as 2 years (Kaunitz 1998) because small residual serum concentrations of MPA may be enough to inhibit a mid-cycle luteinizing hormone surge. Clomiphene citrate may help in these cases.

The mean time to conception after the use of depot progestogens is 9.2 months

Depot progestogen injections are not suitable for couples who wish to conceive within 2 years but women who have used removable rods such as Norplant have been shown to have normal cumulative pregnancy rates after removal (Affendi et al. 1987).

Salpingitis

The choice of contraceptive method has an influence both on the chances of contracting salpingitis and on the severity of the infection.

Fallopian tube damage is the most common acquired form of subfertility, being responsible for about 20% of all cases. It is virtually always caused by sexually acquired infection ascending via the cervix. *Chlamydia trachomatis* is the most common infective agent and is often symptomless so that in 60% of cases of bilateral tubal occlusion there is no previous history of pelvic inflammatory disease.

The risk of subfertility after salpingitis varies according to the severity of infection, the number of attacks and the age of the woman. The risk is said to be 12.8% after a single attack, 35.5% after two attacks and 75% after three or more attacks (Westrom 1975). A mild attack leads to tubal damage in 9.5% of cases but this increases to 20% for a moderately severe attack and 32.1% after a single severe attack.

Cervical mucus is thickened by progestogens and this probably reduces the risk of ascending infection for women choosing hormonal contraception. Pathogenic organisms have been shown to be capable of attaching to the tails of sperm and 'hitching a ride' to reach the upper genital tract. Hence, partners of azoospermic men are said to have a low incidence of pelvic inflammatory disease (Toth et al. 1984).

Even though oestrogens make cervical mucus more penetrable, the overall effect of the combined pill on cervical mucus is usually to make it thicker and less penetrable. Combined oral contraception is said to reduce the risk of pelvic infection by about 50%.

If a woman contracts a pelvic infection while wearing an intrauterine contraceptive device (IUCD) the severity of the infection is increased. This means that hospital admission for pelvic infection is more common for women using an IUCD than for women using other forms of contraception. The IUCD does not cause the infection unless, of course, pathogenic organisms are introduced at the time of insertion.

The levonorgestrel-releasing intrauterine system (IUS) may reduce the risk of pelvic infection by its action on cervical mucus.

Barrier methods provide the best protection from sexually transmitted diseases although the protection is by no means absolute and contraceptive efficacy is lower than other methods. The practice of using pills to minimize conception and barriers to minimize sexually transmitted disease is to be encouraged. The greater the surface covered by the barrier the greater will be the protective effect. Female condoms are therefore thought to be superior to male condoms, which are thought to be better than caps.

Unwanted pregnancies lead to abortion and hence the possibility of postabortal infection and subsequent tubal damage. Despite this risk many studies have failed to show an overall risk of subfertility following termination of pregnancy (e.g. WHO 1984). The risk of infection is at least halved by the use of prophylactic antibiotics. Figures are only available from countries where abortion is legal; illegal abortion has a much higher morbidity.

Ectopic pregnancy

Any effective contraceptive method will lower the risk of ectopic pregnancy and hence the risk of subsequent tubal damage.

If a woman conceives despite the presence of an IUCD the pregnancy is more likely to be ectopic than if she had conceived without one. This is not the same as saying that she is more likely to have an ectopic pregnancy, only that the proportion of intrauterine to ectopic pregnancies is altered. The quoted mechanism for this is that the local inflammatory-like action of the IUCD is greatest close to where the device lies within the uterine cavity and gradually diminishes with increasing distance down the fallopian tubes. Implantation is still inhibited in the tube, but to a lesser degree.

The best example of this is the levonorgestrel IUS. Although up to 25% of the pregnancies occurring with this device *in situ* are ectopic, the overall pregnancy rate is of the order of 0.25 per 1000 women years. This results in a 90% reduction in the expected ectopic pregnancy rate for women not using contraception (Sivin 1998).

The figures are similar for failures after sterilization. The US collaborative survey recorded one-third of all such pregnancies to be ectopic but the 10-year failure rate was only in the region of 4% (Peterson et al. 1996).

The first IVF pregnancy was a tubal pregnancy. It is surprising that IVF pregnancies have a much higher chance of being ectopic (about 5%) than naturally conceived pregnancies considering the fact that the embryos are transferred directly into the uterine cavity. This is probably because the physical stimulation of transfer enhances subendometrial contractions, which transport the embryos through the uterotubal junction. It may be appropriate in some cases to apply clips to the fallopian tubes immediately adjacent to the uterus before attempting IVF so as to avoid this potentially dangerous complication.

Five per cent of IVF pregnancies are ectopic

Other effects

The growth of uterine fibroids is inhibited in women who have used combined pills for long periods (Ross et al. 1986). Fibroids are commonly associated with subfertility although they are rarely the major cause. They may distort the uterine cavity and interfere with implantation or increase the risk of miscarriage. Alternatively they may block the intramural part of the fallopian tube.

Normal cumulative pregnancy rates have been recorded in populations of women immediately after stopping combined oral contraception and after the removal of levonorgestrel implants, copper IUCDs and the levonorgestrel IUS. There also appears to be no delay to fertility after use of progestogen-only pills or contraceptive vaginal rings.

Managing subfertility

Generally speaking the causes of fertility can be divided into five main groups (*Figure 5*). If perfect treatment is provided we should hope to obtain a pregnancy rate equivalent to the natural conception rate, i.e. 1 in 3 per treatment cycle. This is true for ovulation induction in cases of anovulation and for most couples treated with IVF.

The first aim of management is to educate the couple about their fertility and to estimate their chances of natural conception based on their history and on the results of basic tests of ovulation, fallopian tube patency and sperm function. One example might be a couple with normal baseline tests (so-called unexplained subfertility) who have been trying to conceive for 2 years and where the female partner is 31 years old. In this case a reasonable estimate of the chances of normal conception would be in the region of 1 in 50 per month of trying during the next 2 years (Hull 1992).

The failure rate of male condoms can be as high as 1 in 50 and this is usually regarded as too high a risk for couples who definitely wish to avoid pregnancy. Just because our couple are subfertile does not mean that they should risk not using contraception at times when they would prefer to avoid pregnancy, such as the first few months of a new job.

Condom failure rates are equivalent to natural pregnancy rates for many subfertile couples

What is important is that the couple should continue to receive appropriate information and support whether they are trying to conceive or not. Unfortunately different health-care professionals and even different

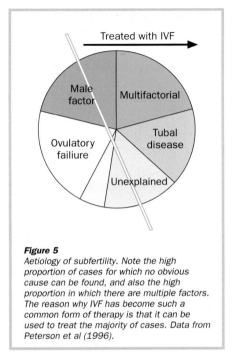

Figure 5
Aetiology of subfertility. Note the high proportion of cases for which no obvious cause can be found, and also the high proportion in which there are multiple factors. The reason why IVF has become such a common form of therapy is that it can be used to treat the majority of cases. Data from Peterson et al (1996).

health-care systems tend to be involved in these two very similar medical problems.

Unusual situations requiring contraception

During investigation

Methods of tubal patency testing hold a risk for a very early pregnancy should they be performed in the second half of the ovarian cycle. This is greatest for an X-ray hysterosalpingogram and least for an ultrasound assessment of tubal patency. These procedures are usually performed exclusively in the follicular phase of the cycle, or alternatively a highly sensitive pregnancy test is performed immediately prior to their use.

During treatment

There are a number of situations where natural conception should be avoided during fertility treatment. One example is when an anovulatory woman undergoes ovulation induction and the ovarian response is greater than expected. Three, four or more pre-ovulatory sized follicles may develop and if conception were to occur there would be a risk of supermultiple gestation. This is seen particularly in women with polycystic ovaries, and all the famous cases publicized in the lay press have been women who have over-responded owing to this condition. It is not possible to predict the time of ovulation and contraceptive precautions need to be taken until the next endometrial bleed. Total abstinence or barrier methods are usually advised, although compliance with these strategies may be poor, particularly in a couple desperate to conceive and unpractised at barrier methods.

Another example is during IVF therapy in cases where there is tubal patency and an adequate sperm count. After oocyte capture some oocytes may remain and there is the risk that conception may occur in vivo as well as in vitro and lead to a supermultiple gestation.

Between treatment cycles

There are all sorts of situations where a couple might wish to avoid conception with certainty for a short period between cycles of fertility treatment. Barrier methods are most popular but oral contraception may be more appropriate for longer periods or if there is a wish for the future treatment cycle to start on a given date. In this case the timing of the withdrawal bleed can be adjusted by oral contraceptive pill intake. There are even occasions when extended downregulation with gonadotrophin releasing hormone superagonists prior to IVF for endometriosis might be extended to allow a conception-free interval prior to therapy.

After treatment

Couples who have spent may years trying to conceive have, not uncommonly, delayed medical treatment for other conditions because of the effect treatment would have had on their fertility. Examples are endometriosis, fibroids, pelvic pain and menorrhagia. The decision to discontinue fertility treatment, whether this has been successful or not, may therefore trigger surprising requests for hysterectomy. It is as if the couple find comfort in the absolute certainty of hysterectomy after many years of having to contend with the uncertain outcome of each cycle of fertility treatment.

Case histories

Case 1

Tanya, a 21-year-old student complains that since stopping her combined pill 3 months ago she has not menstruated. She is studying hard for her final examinations and does not want the added anxiety of a probable gynaecological problem to distract her from her work.

'I've enough on my plate at the moment,' she moans.

Her BMI is 20 and physical examination is normal. She is anxious but clinically euthyroid. A urinary pregnancy test is negative. Her FSH is 3.8 IU/l, LH 3.1 IU/l and prolactin 357 mIU/l.

She is reassured strongly that once the anxiety of her exams is over she will almost certainly begin to menstruate normally again. She is told this may happen again at other times of stress in her life and will do her no harm, but she should not think that she no longer requires contraception.

Case 2

Adele, a 31-year-old woman, asks for advice about foreign travel as she and her husband are planning to work for a charity in central Africa for the next 2 years. After the usual advice about vaccinations and avoiding local endemic disease it transpires that she has not used any form of contraception for the last 5 years but was only pregnant once 3 years ago. This pregnancy proved to be ectopic, requiring right salpingectomy. Her left tube is thought to be damaged but patent.

'I really don't think I'll need any form of contraception, will I?' she says.

The fact that she is not totally infertile is stressed to her. Most hazardous would be a second ectopic pregnancy occurring in a place where urgent medical facilities might not be readily available. An IUCD is relatively contraindicated in the presence of pelvic infection. She is fitted with Norplant.

References

Affendi B, Santoso SS, Djajadilaga et al. (1987) Pregnancy after removal of Norplant implant contraceptive. *Contraception* **36**(2): 203–9.

De Mouzon J, Rossin-Amar B, Bachelot A, Renon C, Devecchi A (1998) [FIVNAT. Influence of attempt rank in in vitro fertilization.] *Contracept Fertil Sexual* **27**(7–8): 466–72.

Dor J, Seidman DS, Ben-Shlomo I, et al. (1996) Cumulative pregnancy rate following in vitro fertilization: the significance of age and infertility aetiology. *Hum Reprod* **11**(2): 425–8.

Fraser IS, Dennerstein GJ (1994) Depo-Provera use in an Australian metropolitan practice. *Med J Aust* **160**(9): 553–6.

Guzick DS, Wilkes C, Jones HW (1986) Cumulative pregnancy rates for in vitro fertilization. *Fertil Steril* **46**(4): 663–7.

Hull MG (1992) Infertility treatment; relative effectiveness of conventional and assisted conception methods. *Hum Reprod* **7**: 785–96.

Hull MG, Bromham DR, Savage PE, Jackson JA, Jacobs HS (1981) Normal fertility in women with post pill amenorrhoea. *Lancet* **i**(8234): 1329–32.

Jones WR (1977) Post-pill amenorrhoea—how much of a problem? *Austral Fam Phys* (suppl): 16–18.

Kaunitz AM (1998) Injectable depot medroxyprogesterone acetate contraception: an update for US clinicians. *Int J Fertil Wom Med* **43**(2): 73–83.

Mishell DR (1996) Pharmacokinetics of depot medroxyprogesterone acetate contraception. *J Reprod Med* **41**(5 suppl): 381–90.

Peterson HB, Xia Z, Hughes JM, et al. (1996) The risk of pregnancy after tubal sterilization: findings from the US Collaborative Review of Sterilization. *Am J Obstet Gynecol* **174**: 1161–70.

Ross RF, Pike MC, Vessey MP et al. (1986) Risk factors for uterine fibroids: reduced risk associated with oral contraception. *Br Med J* **293**: 359–63.

Sivin I (1998) Potential benefits in developing countries through use of the levonorgestrel-releasing intrauterine system. *Gynaecol Forum* **3**(3): 23–5.

Toth A, Lesser ML, Labriola D (1984) The development of infections of the genitourinary tract in the wives of infertile males and the possible role of spermatozoa in the development of salpingitis. *Surg Gynecol Obstet* **159**(6): 565–9.

Weisberg W (1982) Fertility after discontinuation of oral contraceptives. *Clin Reprod Fertil* **1**(4): 261–72.

Westrom L (1975) Effect of acute pelvic inflammatory disease on fertility. *Am J Obstet Gynecol* **121**(5): 707–13.

WHO (1984) Secondary infertility following induced abortion. *Stud Fam Plan* **15**(6 pt 1): 291–5.

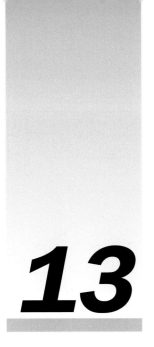

Women with migraine

Anne MacGregor

13

Migraine is the most common cause of severe episodic recurrent headache. Attacks typically last 4–72 hours and can occur, on average, every 4–6 weeks. Although migraine is a benign condition, the severity and frequency of attacks can result in significant disability and reduced quality of life, even between attacks (Osterhaus et al. 1994). During attacks, symptoms of heightened sensitivity to light, sound and smell, accompanied by nausea, vomiting and general malaise, can be more distressing to the patient than the headache itself.

The first migraine attack occurs before the age of 40 years in 90% of cases

The first attack of migraine usually occurs during the teens and early twenties, with 90% of attacks occurring before age 40 years (Selby and Lance 1960). Migraine typically disappears after the age of 50 years (Blau 1987a). Lifetime prevalence of migraine has been shown to be 8% in men and 25% in women (Rasmussen et al. 1991). Prevalence varies by age, increasing from menarche to about age 42 years and declining thereafter (Stewart et al. 1994). The changing hormonal environment in women is considered to be the main reason for the increased female prevalence during the reproductive years, with varying improvement or deterioration associated with menstruation, use of hormonal contraception, pregnancy, the menopause and use of hormone replacement therapy.

The two most frequently encountered types of migraine differ only in the presence or absence of an 'aura'. About 70–80% of migraineurs experience attacks of migraine without aura (formerly known as common or simple migraine); 10% have migraine with aura (formerly known as classical or focal migraine); 15–20% have both types of attack. Less than 1% of attacks are of aura alone, with no ensuing headache.

Clinically, an attack of migraine can further be divided into five distinct phases (Blau 1987b) as shown in *Figure 1*.

1. *Prodromal/premonitory phase*: not all migraineurs are aware of prodromal symptoms, which can precede attacks of both migraine with and without aura by

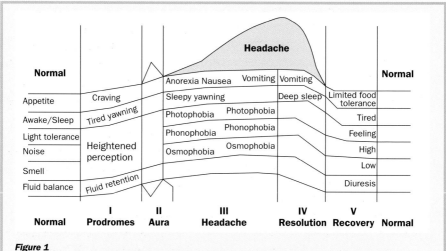

Figure 1
Symptoms and signs during phases of complete classic migraine attacks. Reproduced with permission from Blau JN (1992) Migraine: theories of pathogenesis. Lancet **339**: *1202–7.*

12–24 hours. Symptoms are suggestive of hypothalamic disturbance and are distinct from, and unrelated to, the aura. They include irritability, feeling 'high' or 'low'; extreme lethargy and yawning; dysphasia; anorexia, constipation or diarrhoea; urinary frequency, thirst or fluid retention. Friends, family or work colleagues are more likely to notice these symptoms than the patient. Some prodromal symptoms are incorrectly blamed as triggers for the attack. For example, craving for sweet foods may result in a desire to eat chocolate. A few people feel 'on top of the world' before an attack and rush around, later thinking that the attack was caused by overactivity. In fact, these are signs that the attack has already begun. Recognition of these prodromal symptoms can be of enormous benefit since avoiding known trigger factors during this time may be all that is necessary to stop the attack developing further.

2. *Aura* (when present): symptoms of aura probably arise from the cerebral cortex or brain stem and gradually develop over 5–20 minutes, last under 1 hour, and usually completely resolve before the onset of headache. Atypical or permanent symptoms warrant further investigation. Homonymous visual symptoms are most common, experienced in 99% of auras (Russell and Olesen 1996). Sensory disturbance is less common (31%) and is usually associated with visual symptoms. Speech disturbance and motor symptoms can also be present (18% and 6%, respectively) but only in association with visual and/or sensory symptoms. Symptoms usually follow one another in succession beginning with visual symptoms, followed by sensory symptoms, dysphasia and weakness.

About 20–30% of migraine attacks are accompanied by aura

3. *Headache and associated symptoms*: the throbbing headache is typically unilateral, sometimes swapping sides during an attack, but may be bilateral. It is aggravated by movement of the head and accompanied by nausea or vomiting, photophobia and/or phonophobia. Although some patients can continue limited activities, many have to retire to bed in a darkened room until symptoms subside.

4. *Resolution*: other than with effective medication, the natural course of migraine is to resolve with sleep (Wilkinson et al. 1978). Some attacks, particularly in children, improve after vomiting.

5. *Recovery* (postdromal phase): after the headache has gone most migraineurs feel drained and 'washed out' for a further day. Rarely, they feel energetic and even euphoric.

Diagnosing migraine

Because the diagnosis of migraine is frequently confused with other headaches, the International Headache Society (IHS) published a comprehensive headache classification (Headache Classification Committee of the IHS 1988). However, the criteria are not suited to routine clinical use.

Standard texts provide examples of how to diagnose migraine by history and examination (British Association for the Study of Headache 1999, MacGregor 1999a). Most cases can be identified by a positive response to the following questions: 'Have you ever had a migraine?' 'Have you ever had a headache accompanied by nausea?' 'Have you ever had a severe headache accompanied by hypersensitivity to light and sound?' (Gervil et al. 1988). The attacks will last 1–3 days with complete freedom from symptoms between attacks. Daily headaches are not migraine, although migraine and daily headaches may coexist. Aura can be identified by a positive response to the question 'Have you ever had visual disturbances lasting 5–60 minutes followed by headache?' (Gervil et al. 1998).

Aura or TIA?

Doctors are often concerned about distinguishing between transient ischaemic attacks (TIA) and migraine aura (*Table 1*). It is necessary to take a careful history to ensure symptoms are typical of migraine. Fortunately, certain features of the migraine aura can help distinguish between migraine and the focal neurological symptoms of cerebral ischaemia. Some patients find it hard to describe auras. Common mistakes include reports of sudden onset when it is gradual, of monocular disturbances which are homonymous, and incorrect duration of aura (Headache Classification Committee of the IHS 1988). If there is any uncertainty, encourage patients to record their symptoms prospectively.

Progression of symptoms

The evolution of a migraine aura is slow, taking several minutes to spread to maximum distribution. In contrast, the motor and sensory spread of cerebral ischaemia is rapid, taking only seconds to move from the face to the hand, progressing rapidly down the trunk to affect the lower limb.

Symptoms

Visual symptoms of migraine are usually symmetrical, affecting one hemifield of both eyes, although subjectively they may appear to affect only one eye. A migrainous scotoma is

Table 1
Differences between ischaemic episodes and migraine aura.

	TIA	Migraine
History	No previous episodes	Similar attacks in the past (typically migraine onset childhood/early adult)
Onset/progression of symptoms	Sudden (seconds)	Slow evolution over several minutes
Duration	>1 hour	<1 hour (typically 20–30 min)
Timing	Occurs with or without headache, with no temporal relationship	Precedes and resolves before onset of typical migraine headache
Visual symptoms	Monocular, negative (black) scotoma	Present in 99% of auras. Homonymous positive (bright) scotoma gradually enlarging across visual field into 'C' shape with scintillating zigzag edges
Sensory/motor symptoms	May occur without visual symptoms May include leg Negative (limb feels 'dead')	Present in one-third of auras — usually in association with visual symptoms Rarely affects leg Positive ('pins and needles')
Headache	No subsequent headache, or symptoms continue in association with headache	Migraine headache and association symptoms typically follow resolution of aura. Aura may occur without headache, but confirm past history of migraine

From Macgregor (1999b).

TIA, transient ischaemic attack.

typically positive (bright), starting as a small spot gradually increasing in size to assume the shape of a letter C, developing scintillating edges which appear as zigzags or 'fortifications'—a term coined in the late eighteenth century because the visual disturbances resembled a fortified town surrounded by bastions. The aura usually starts at or near the centre of fixation, gradually spreading laterally, increasing in size over a period of 5–30 minutes. In contrast, thrombotic symptoms do not generally have the scintillating and spreading features of the visual aura of migraine and the visual loss usually described as a monocular negative scotoma (black). Transient monocular blindness is *not* typical of migraine and prompts urgent investigation. Generalized 'spots before the eyes', 'flashing lights', blurring of vision, photophobia affecting the whole visual field of both eyes and of variable duration before or with headache often occur during migraine and are not suggestive of focal ischaemia.

Transient monocular blindness is not typical of migraine and prompts urgent investigation

Sensory symptoms are positive, i.e. a sensation of pins and needles rather than numbness. In an ischaemic episode, a sense of numbness or 'deadness' is described. Migraine symptoms have a characteristic unilateral distribution affecting one arm, often spreading over several minutes proximally from the hand to affect the mouth and tongue (cheiro-oral

distribution). The leg is rarely affected in migraine.

History of symptoms

Migraine auras usually follow a similar pattern with each attack although the duration of aura may alter. Therefore, a long history of similar attacks, particularly if onset is in childhood or early adult life, is reassuring. If aura symptoms suddenly change, further investigation may be warranted.

Treating migraine

The treatment of migraine in women using hormonal contraception is the same as that recommended for women using other methods of, or not using, contraception. Acute treatment regimens usually include a combination of analgesics with or without prokinetic antiemetics, non-steroidal anti-inflammatory drugs, ergot derivatives and triptans (British Association for the Study of Headache 1999). In the UK, ergots are contraindicated in women using combined oral contraceptives (COCs) (see below). Commonly used prophylactic treatments have no pharmacokinetic interactions with COCs.

Combined oral contraceptives

Effects on migraine

Headache is a common side-effect of COC use, with initial exacerbation in the early cycles of use followed by resolution with continued use (Slugge and Lawson 1967). The frequency of headache may depend on the type of progestogen and the dose of oestrogen used. Studies of COCs containing levonorgestrel, a second-generation progestogen, note headache in approximately 10% of all cycles (Guillebaud 1983). In contrast, COCs containing third-generation progestogens appear to have less associated headache. A review of studies using a COC containing 30 μg ethinyloestradiol and 150 μg desogestrel found headache to affect only 5% of women during the sixth cycle (Fotherby 1998). A review of studies using only 20 μg ethinyloestradiol and 150 μg desogestrel noted a headache incidence of less than 2% by the sixth cycle (Fotherby 1992).

The effect of COCs on migraine is extremely variable. It is important to note that in a significant proportion of women migraine improves, and many report no change in migraine frequency or severity. Many women experience migraine attacks during the pill-free interval of COCs (Dalton 1976). Of concern are those women whose migraine becomes more frequent or severe and those who develop migraine for the first time soon after starting COCs, particularly if the attacks are migraine with aura. These women appear to be at increased risk of ischaemic stroke.

Possible mechanisms of increased migraine in COC users

Little research has been undertaken on the possible mechanisms for the adverse changes in migraine associated with COC use. With regard to aura, Mazal (1978) reported a case of a woman who developed migraine with aura after starting COCs associated with increased platelet aggregation. Improvement after ceasing COCs was related to a gradual return to normal platelet activity. Similarly, Hanington et al. (1982) studied women who developed migraine with aura after starting COCs and women who reported exacerbation of pre-existing aura. They noted increased platelet aggregation to serotonin in both groups, which declined with the cessation of COCs over 4–6 months, paralleling a gradual improvement in migraine. Platelet aggregation has been implicated in aura owing to the production of platelet microemboli in pial vessels of the visual cortex (Peatfield 1987). The mechanism of attacks in association with the falling hormone levels occurring during the pill-free interval is probably similar to one recognized mechanism of 'menstrual' migraine, i.e. oestrogen withdrawal (Somerville 1975). Such attacks are typically migraine without aura.

Migraine, COCs and risk of ischaemic stroke

Use of COCs is an established risk factor for ischaemic stroke (*Table 2*) although the absolute risk is very small because the incidence of ischaemic stroke is very low in young women (WHO 1996a). High-dose oestrogen pills carry a higher risk than low-dose oestrogen pills. There appears to be no difference between the risk of ischaemic stroke in users of second- and third-generation progestogens (Heinemann et al. 1997).

The Collaborative Group for the Study of Stroke in Young Women (CGSS 1975) were the first to identify an increased risk of stroke in COC users with migraine. Lidegaard (1993) studied 794 women aged 15–44 years in Denmark (population 5.2 million) who suffered a cerebral thromboembolic attack in 1985–9 and age-matched randomly selected controls. He reported significant odds ratios (OR) of 2.9 for stroke in users of COCs containing 50 µg of synthetic ethinyloestradiol, 1.8 for COCs containing 30–40 µg of ethinyloestradiol, but no excess risk (OR 0.9) for progestogen-only pills (POPs). In 1995 Lidegaard reported, from the same data base, an OR of 2.8 for migraine (of any variety occurring more than once a month), with an apparent multiplicative effect between migraine, COC use and smoking (Lidegaard 1995). For women with migraine taking COCs, the OR was 5.

Smoking significantly increases the risk of ischaemic stroke in migraine sufferers taking the COC

Tzourio et al. (1993) found a significant increased risk (OR 4.3) of ischaemic stroke in migraine with and without aura among women under the age of 45 years, rising to an odds ratio of 10.2 if they smoked. A later paper by the same workers (Tzourio et al. 1995) reported significant ORs of 3.0 in migraine without aura, 6.2 for migraine with aura, and 13.9 for all migraineurs who took oral contraceptives. They did not report the COC risk separately for each type of migraine.

Carolei et al. (1996) reported on several risk factors for cerebral ischaemia in 308 men and women aged 15–44 years with a history of stroke or transient ischaemic attacks compared with a control population. Use of COCs was associated with an OR for ischaemic stroke of 1.8. A history of migraine was found to be an independent risk factor with a crude OR of 8.6 for migraine with aura compared with 1.0 for migraine without aura. Subgroup analysis of women under the age of 35 years identified migraine to be the only significant risk factor for cerebral ischaemia for that group, with a crude

Table 2
Odds ratios for ischaemic stroke.

	OR migraine (95% CI) [no. cases/controls]	Ethinyloestradiol dose (µg)	OR COC use (95% CI) [no. cases/controls]	OR COC use plus migraine^a (95% CI) [no. cases/controls]
CGSS (1975)	**2.0 RR**^b (1.2–3.3) [30/113]	≥50	**4.9 RR** (2.9–8.3) [41/38]	**5.9 RR** (2.9–12.2) [18/15]
Tzourio et al. (1995)	**3.5** (1.8–6.4) [43/52] with or without aura^c	All doses	**3.1** (1.2–8.2)	**13.9** (5.5–35.1)
	3.0 (1.5–5.8) [33/42] without aura^c	50	**4.8**	–
	6.2 (2.1–18.0) [10/10] with aura^c	30–40	**2.7**	–
		20	**1.7**	–
Lidegaard (1993, 1995)	**2.8** with or without aura^d	All doses	–	5
		50	**2.9** (1.6–5.4)	–
		30–40	**1.8** (1.1–2.9)	–
Carolei et al. (1996)	**1.3** with or without aura^c (0.7–2.4)	All doses	**1.3** (0.6–2.6) [14/21]	No data
	3.7 (1.5–9.0) if <35 yr with aura			
	8.6 (1–75) with aura			
	1.0 (0.5–2.0) without aura			
WHO (1996a)	No data	All doses (Europe)	**2.24** (1.31–3.82) [52/87]	No data
		≥50	**5.3** (2.56–11.0) [32/35]	
		<50	**1.53** (0.71–3.31) [20/52]	
Chang et al. (1999)	**2.97** (0.66–13.5) [7/9] without aura^c	All doses	**2.76** (1.01–7.55) [19/42]	**16.9** (2.72–106) [10/3]
	3.81 (1.26–11.5) [19/17] with aura^c	≥50	**7.95** (1.94–32.6) [9/14]	Cannot be calculated
		<50	**1.19** (0.33–4.29) [10/28]	**6.59** (0.79–54.8) [4/3]

From MacGregor (1999b).

CI, confidence interval; COC, combined oral contraceptive; OR, odds ratio; RR, relative risk.

^a Data not differentiated for type of migraine

^b Diagnosis based on presence of two or more of the following symptoms: unilateral headache, throbbing quality, visual scintillation, vomiting and other symptoms (study predates IHS criteria).

^c Diagnosis made using IHS criteria.

^d Self-reported diagnosis; attack frequency >1 per month.

OR of 3.7. Once again they did not study the combined effect of COCs and migraine.

More recently, Chang et al. (1999) published a case–control study of self-reported headache in 291 women aged 20–44 years. The OR for ischaemic stroke was 2.97 in women with migraine without aura and 3.81 in migraine with aura. Since their data included women who may have had a distant past history of a single attack with aura, the real risk associated with aura is difficult to interpret. Further, the definition of aura used may not have been sufficiently sensitive so that cases of prodromal symptoms could have been included in the 'aura' group. However, this study highlighted the synergistic effects of multiple risk factors

with an OR of 34.4 for ischaemic stroke in migraineurs who smoke and use COCs.

Becker (1997) calculated the risks in relation to the expected incidence of ischaemic stroke per 100 000 women per year (*Figure 2*). According to his figures, 28 per 100 000 COC users with migraine with aura would expect an ischaemic stroke. This does not consider the synergistic effects of additional risk factors, particularly smoking. This figure compares to an expected stroke incidence of 8.1 per 100 000 pregnancies (Kittner et al. 1996).

Migraine aura can be associated with two events that may contribute to increased risk of

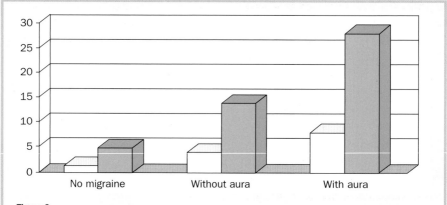

Figure 2
Expected incidence of ischaemic stroke per 100 000 women per year aged 25–34 years, based on data from Becker (1997). From MacGregor (1999b). Shaded bars, COC users; white bars, non-users.

ischaemic stroke. Firstly, reduced cerebral blood flow is known to occur during migraine aura (Goadsby 1997). This is probably of significance in stroke arising during an attack of migraine (Chang et al. 1999). Secondly, increased platelet aggregation, a recognized risk factor for ischaemic stroke, has been reported in migraine (Kalendovsky et al. 1975, Couch and Hassanein 1977, Gawel and Rose 1982) particularly when aura develops in association with COC use (Mazal 1978, Hanington et al. 1982).

Progestogen-only methods

Effects on migraine

Few studies differentiate between headache and migraine, most citing incidence of headache only. Consequently, adverse events reporting headache will include migraine. Since the studies do not compare with placebo (for obvious reasons), the true effect of progestogen-only methods is not clear. In women not using hormonal contraception, a recognized trigger of 'menstrual' migraine is oestrogen withdrawal in the late luteal phase of the menstrual cycle (Somerville 1975). Somerville also noted a close relationship between migraine and uterine bleeding, even when ovulation was suppressed (Somerville 1970). Although Somerville suggested that this may be due to fluctuations in oestrogen levels, prostaglandins have also been

implicated (Benedetto et al. 1997), levels of which increase three-fold in the uterine endometrium during the luteal phase with a further increase during menstruation (Speroff et al. 1994). Since most progestogen-only methods, with the exception of injectable progestogens, do not entirely abolish the ovarian cycle but often disrupt it, hormonal triggers of migraine remain. Even when ovulation is suppressed, fluctuations in oestrogen levels can still occur (Shearman 1964) so that oestrogen withdrawal will still act as a migraine trigger (Somerville 1970). This occurs less with injectable contraceptives, which can inhibit the ovarian cycle and induce amenorrhoea, achieving improvement in migraine (Somerville 1970).

Progestogen-only pill

A MEDLINE search did not reveal any published studies of headache associated with use of the progestogen-only pill, although it is a recognized side-effect (Schering, data on file). Anecdotally, headache and migraine are more likely to improve in women who become amenorrhoeic, probably for the reasons discussed above.

Subdermal implants

Aside from menstrual irregularity, headache is the main reason reported for discontinuing use of levonorgestrel implants (Norplant).

Headaches have been noted in 25–50% of women using Norplant (Darney et al 1990, Cullins 1993) with headache given as the reason for discontinuation in 1.3% (Croshy et al. 1993). Studies with Implanon, the new single-rod implant, report headache to be in most common drug-related adverse event, affecting 7% of women (Kiriwat et al. 1998). Headache was given as the reason for discontinuation in 0.5% of women on Implanon compared with 0.3% of women on Norplant (Edwards and Moore 1999).

Depot progestogens

Two studies have shown increase in headache reported over time with both depot medroxyprogesterone acetate (DMPA) and norethisterone enanthate (NET-EN). A World Health Organization study (WHO 1978) reported more frequent headache in DMPA users (10.7%) than with NET-EN subjects (6.9%), a difference that was statistically significant. Furthermore, there was a consistent increase in the proportion of DMPA subjects complaining of headache, from 8.5% during the first visit to 15.7% during the fourth visit ($P < 0.01$). No comparable increase was observed in NET-EN users.

Similar results for DMPA were reported in a later study by Salem et al. (1988). Among DMPA users, headache was reported in 11.6% of users at 3 months and 15% at 12 months. An increase over time was also seen among NET-EN users, with headache reported in 3.2% of users at 3 months and 19.4% at 12 months.

As with all methods of contraception, further work is needed to assess the differential effect on headache and migraine. Studies suggest that continued use of DMPA may have a beneficial effect on 'menstrual' migraine, probably related to inhibition of ovulation, loss of ovarian cycle and resultant amenorrhoea (MacGregor EA, unpublished observations).

Levonorgestrel-releasing intrauterine system

Headache is a common complaint in early months of use of the levonorgestrel-releasing intrauterine system (LNG IUS), but settles with continued use. Andersson et al. (1994) reported a 2.8% incidence of headache in LNG IUS users 3 months after insertion compared with 0.8% in users of Nova-T, a copper device. By 60 months of use, headache in LNG IUS users had fallen to 1.6% compared with 1% in Nova-T users.

Migraine, progestogens and risk of ischaemic stroke

There is no evidence that use of progestogen-only contraception is associated with an increased risk of ischaemic stroke (Fotherby

1989, Fahmy et al. 1991, Lidegaard 1993, Samsioe 1994, Tzourio et al. 1995, WHO 1998).

Non-hormonal methods

Headache is reported as an adverse event in trials of non-hormonal methods, which is not surprising since headache and migraine are a common complaint in all women. Anecdotally, 'menstrual' headache is more common in women with dysmenorrhoea and menorrhagia, which occur in association with copper intrauterine devices.

Clinical practice: prescribing contraception to women with migraine

Most women with headaches or migraine can choose whichever contraceptive method meets their needs. Although headaches may worsen soon after starting hormonal contraception, women can be reassured that these are likely to settle with continued use of their chosen contraceptive method.

However, specific advice is necessary for women with migraine who choose to use COCs in order to minimize the risk of ischaemic stroke. The absolute risk of ischaemic stroke is very low in otherwise healthy young women, and since COCs currently used contain low doses of

ethinyloestradiol, their use is associated with a minimally increased risk. Therefore, for the majority of women, migraine itself is not a contraindication to COC use. However, the presence of certain factors may sufficiently increase the risk of ischaemic stroke to justify withholding COCs in favour of alternative methods of contraception (MacGregor and Guillebaud 1998). Recommendations are shown in *Figure 3*. The World Health Organization categories (see Chapter 4) for initiating and continuing use of contraceptive methods are included in these recommendations (WHO 1996b).

Advantages of COC use outweigh disadvantages (WHO category 2)

Ethinyloestradiol contraception may be given with regular supervision and reassessment of risk factors in the following cases. The women should be counselled to seek medical advice should any adverse change in her migraine occur, and to contact a doctor as soon as possible if focal symptoms suggestive of aura or cerebral ischaemia develop.

Migraine without aura in a woman who has no additional risk factors for stroke

Although data are limited, migraine without aura, in the absence of other risk factors for

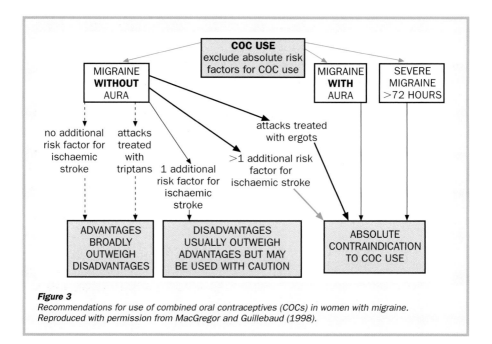

Figure 3
Recommendations for use of combined oral contraceptives (COCs) in women with migraine. Reproduced with permission from MacGregor and Guillebaud (1998).

stroke, carries a small but significant increased risk of ischaemic stroke. Women with migraine without aura using COCs should have regular reassessment of arterial risk factors. Increased frequency of migraine may be associated with increased risk of stroke, and withdrawal of COCs should be considered (Bickerstaff 1975).

Women with migraine without aura using COCs should be regularly assessed for arterial risk factors

Concurrent use of 'triptans'

Naratriptan, rizatriptan, sumatriptan and zolmitriptan have been evaluated for the treatment of migraine in clinical trials. Since effective contraception was a prerequisite to inclusion in these studies, many women were taking COCs. To date, no relevant interactions or adverse events have been associated with the co-administration of 'triptans' and COCs. Reference should be made to the data sheets for full prescribing details of each 'triptan'.

Disadvantages of COC use usually outweigh the advantages but COCs may be used with caution (WHO category 3)

Migraine without aura in a woman who has one additional risk factor for stroke that is not in itself an absolute contraindication to COC use

The presence of additional risk factors, particularly smoking, increases the risk of cerebral ischaemia in women with migraine using COCs (Tzourio et al. 1993, Chang et al. 1999). Women should be advised to stop smoking. However, COCs may be used with caution with regular assessment of other risk factors for stroke, such as hypertension, diabetes and obesity, and with counselling about adverse changes in migraine symptoms and frequency.

Absolute contraindications to COC use (WHO category 4)

Although use of COCs is acceptable in the majority of women with migraine, there are some types of migraine which absolutely contraindicate the use of COCs. Such attacks may be pre-existing or occur for the first time in a pill-taker. In a woman with pre-existing migraine without aura, any adverse change in the pattern of migraine (increased frequency, increased duration, onset of aura), development of severe and/or more frequent non-migraine headache, or development of focal neurological symptoms should prompt discontinuation of COCs. The woman should be investigated or referred, as appropriate, to rule out cerebrovascular events.

Migraine with aura

Until further data are available, COCs should be contraindicated for use in migraine with aura. This is based on the evidence that the risk of ischaemic stroke in women with aura using COCs is greater than the risk of ischaemic stroke associated with pregnancy. These women are not denied effective contraception, as several alternative methods now available are as—if not more—effective than COCs.

A woman experiencing focal neurological symptoms should be transferred immediately, even during an attack, to a method of contraception that does not contain ethinyloestradiol. She should be warned that she may continue to get migraine with or without aura but there would no longer be the added concern that her contraception would amplify the small risk of stroke.

Migraine without aura in a woman who has more than one additional risk factor for stroke

The presence of more than one risk factor is associated with an unacceptable increased risk of thrombotic stroke due to a synergistic effect (Chang et al. 1999). Therefore, non-ethinyloestradiol contraception is recommended for women with multiple risk factors.

Severe migraine, even in the absence of underlying organic disease, is an absolute contraindication for ethinyloestradiol contraception

Severe migraine and 'status migrainosus'

Severe migraine, formerly known as 'crescendo migraine', means any migraine sustained for 3 or more days, with or without treatment, while becoming ever more severe, even in the absence of any focal symptoms. 'Status migrainosus' describes attacks of *continuous* headache lasting more than 72 hours, often related to medication misuse from the chronic (typically daily) use of acute headache treatments such as analgesics and/or ergot derivatives (Couch and Diamond 1983). Since it may be difficult to distinguish clearly between severe migraine and organic cerebral ischaemia, the presence of such attacks absolutely contraindicates COCs until appropriate investigations exclude underlying disease. Severe migraine, even in the absence of underlying organic disease, is also an absolute contraindication for use of ethinyloestradiol contraception. However, if attacks resolve after treatment of medication misuse, the clinician may review the eligibility of the woman for COC use.

Concurrent use of ergot

Ergot alkaloids, including ergotamine and dihydroergotamine, have widespread vasoconstrictor actions and their (mis)use, especially when combined with smoking and COCs, has been associated with arterial thrombosis (Wollersheim et al. 1987).

The occurrence of a woman's first attack of any migraine while taking COCs

The occurrence of a woman's first-ever attack of any migraine (with or without aura) has been specified in manufacturers' data sheets as grounds to discontinue the pill. Certainly, if a woman develops her first attack of migraine *with* aura when using COCs, she should stop the pill immediately. Advice for a woman developing her first attack of migraine *without* aura during COC use is less clear. If there is any concern that the symptoms are associated with a thomboembolic phenomenon, i.e. if other risk factors are apparent, COCs should be discontinued immediately and the symptoms evaluated. Provided that this rare possibility is considered and carefully excluded, and no further problems develop from the first attack, combined pills may be continued or recommenced, with counselling and regular supervision.

A history of episodes of typical migraine with aura

A brief history of such attacks occurring, for example, more than 5 years before commencing COC use, or a history of migraine with aura only during pregnancy, may be regarded as relative contraindications. Combined oral contraception may be given a trial, with counselling and regular supervision. Women should be given a specific warning that

onset of focal neurological symptoms after starting COCs means that they should stop the pill immediately, use alternative contraception, and seek medical advice as soon as possible.

'Ordinary' headaches

'Ordinary' headaches are not a contraindication to COC use as they are more in the nature of a common side-effect for which the woman may seek help. Sometimes changing to a different brand of COC is effective. Women should be advised to seek professional advice if they have any doubts about the nature of any headache.

Migraine in the pill-free week

During the pill-free week levels of oestrogen fall. Migraine occurring during this time appears to be triggered by oestrogen withdrawal, similar to the mechanism of 'menstrual' migraine (Somerville 1975). It should be noted that 'oestrogen withdrawal' migraine is typically *without* aura and therefore of less concern. Once a pattern of migraine linked to the pill-free interval has been established, several options can be tried. The 'tricycle' regimen, i.e. taking three packets without a break, using the lowest acceptable fixed dose formulation, means that the woman has only five such migraines a year instead of 13. Changing the formulation, or addition of a natural oestrogen supplement (as used for oestrogen replacement therapy) during the pill-free interval, may be tried. Consideration should be given to stopping the pill, or changing to non-ethinyloestradiol contraception, if headaches are severe after tricycling or adding natural oestrogen, and certainly if there is any change in symptoms.

Emergency contraception

Pending further data, combined hormonal postcoital contraception is contraindicated for a woman with a past history of migraine with aura presenting *during an attack of migraine* (with or without aura) but not otherwise (Kubba and Wilkinson 1998).

A recent study suggested that the levonorgestrel regimen was better tolerated and more effective than the Yuzpe regimen (Task Force on Postovulatory Methods of Fertility Regulation 1998). Headache was reported in 20.2% of women using Yuzpe with 16.8% using levonorgestrel, a difference that was not significant.

A copper intrauterine device (not the levonorgestrel-releasing IUS) is an effective alternative (Kubba and Wilkinson 1998).

The future

Combined injectable contraceptives are available in some countries and research on combined contraceptive transdermal patches is progressing. Since the dose of oestrogen is much lower in both these methods than with oral preparations, research may show them to be suitable for some women for whom combined oral contraceptives are contraindicated.

Case histories

Case 1

Maureen, a 30-year-old checkout operator, attended her local accident and emergency department on a Sunday evening 24 hours after unprotected sexual intercourse, requesting emergency contraception. She takes sumatriptan for migraine with aura.

'I had to stop the pill because of my bad migraine,' she says. 'So I want the coil.'

The department had no trained personnel on duty to fit an IUCD and Maureen could not attend the next family planning clinic because of work. Her last migraine had ended 3 days earlier so she was reassured that she could safely take combined emergency contraception (PC4). However, because she had been warned to avoid oestrogen-containing contraception she was worried about taking it. She was counselled about progestogen-only emergency contraception and, after convincing her of the greater safety of progestogens, she agreed to take it.

She was given a letter to take to her family planning clinic or her general practitioner and was advised to make an appointment as soon as possible in order to discuss options for long-term contraception. She took the leaflets about different methods of contraception and safe sex.

Case 2

Sheila, 22 years old, visited her general practitioner for a repeat COC prescription. She had been taking the pill for 4 years. Her usual doctor was on maternity leave so she saw a locum. He asked her about her medical history, including headaches. She mentioned that she had been off work a couple of days last month because of migraines. The doctor confirmed they were migraine as she had experienced two attacks of severe headache, which on each occasion lasted most of one day with associated nausea, photophobia and general malaise.

Although she felt very tired before each attack and complained that her vision was blurred, she had no neurological symptoms suggestive of migraine aura or TIA. She stayed in bed for most of the day but was well between attacks. The migraines were not linked to the pill-free week. She had no other medical problems, there was no relevant family history, she was normotensive and her only other risk factor for COC use was that she smoked 10 cigarettes a day.

'I had headaches like this when I was a child, but I haven't had any for ages. My mum gets them really bad. I've had a lot of problems at work recently and put it down to that. I won't have to stop the pill, will I? I really can't risk getting pregnant.'

The doctor gave Sheila a booklet about migraine, which included a list of triggers and a diary card. He warned her that although the risk was extremely small, the combination of taking the pill, smoking and having migraine could increase her risk of a stroke. He strongly advised her to stop smoking as this would greatly reduce the risk. He gave her a repeat COC for 3 months and asked her to keep a record of all her headaches and to identify any triggers. He also gave her leaflets about other methods of contraception, which she should consider if the migraines were continuing and she had not stopped smoking by her next review. She was warned to stop the pill immediately if she experienced any unusual symptoms, such as visual disturbance or weakness of a limb, and to seek medical advice.

References

Andersson K, Odlind V, Rybo G (1994) Levonorgestrel-releasing and copper-releasing (Nova T) IUDs during five years of use: a randomized comparative trial. *Contraception* 49: 56–72.

Becker WJ (1997) Migraine and oral contraceptives. *Can J Neurol Sci* 24: 16–21.

Benedetto C, Allais G, Ciochetto D, De Lorenzo C (1997) Pathophysiological aspects of menstrual migraine. *Cephalalgia* 17(suppl 20): 32–4.

Bickerstaff ER (1975) *Neurological Complications of Oral Contraceptives.* Oxford: Clarendon Press.

Blau JN (1987a) Loss of migraine: when, why and how. *J Roy Coll Phys Lond* 21: 140–2.

Blau JN (1987b) The clinical picture. In: Blau JN (ed.) *Migraine — Clinical, Therapeutic, Conceptual and Research Aspects.* London: Chapman & Hall.

British Association for the Study of Headache (1999) *Guidelines for All Doctors in the Diagnosis and Management of Migraine.* London: BASH, c/o the Princess Margaret Migraine Clinic, Charing Cross Hospital, Fulham Palace Road, London W6 8RF, UK.

Carolei A, Marini C, De Matteis G et al. (1996) History of migraine and risk of cerebral ischaemia in young adults. *Lancet* 347: 1503–6.

[CGSS] Collaborative Group for the Study of Stroke in Young Women (1975) Oral contraceptives and stroke in young women: associated risk factors. *JAMA* 231: 718–22.

Chang CL, Donaghy M, Poulter N et al. (1999) Migraine and stroke in young women: case-control study. *Br Med J* 318: 13–8.

Couch JR, Diamond S (1983) Status migrainosus: causative and therapeutic aspects. *Headache* 23: 64–101.

Couch JR, Hassanein RS (1977) Platelet aggregability in migraine. *Neurology* 27: 843–8.

Croshy UD, Schwarz BE, Gluck KL, Heartwell SE (1993) A preliminary report of Norplant implant insertion in large urban family planning program. *Contraception* 48: 359–66.

Cullins VE (1993) Preliminary experience with Norplant in an inner city population. *Contraception* 47: 193–203.

Dalton K (1976) Migraine and oral contraceptives. *Headache* 15: 247–51.

Darney PD, Atkinson E, Tanner S et al. (1990) Acceptance and perceptions of Norplant users in San Francisco, USA. *Stud Fam Plan* 21: 152–62

Edwards JE, Moore A (1999) Implanon. A review of clinical studies. *Br J Fam Plan* 24: 3–16.

Fahmy K, Khairy M, Allam G, Gobran F, Alloush M (1991) Effect of depo-medroxyprogesterone acetate on coagulation factors and serum lipids in Egyptian women. *Contraception* 44: 431–44.

Fotherby K (1989) The progestogen-only pill and thrombosis. *Br J Fam Plan* 15: 83–5.

Fotherby K (1992) Clinical experience and pharmacological effects of an oral contraceptive containing 20 micrograms oestrogen. *Contraception* 46: 477–88.

Fotherby K (1998) Twelve years of clinical

experience with an oral contraceptive containing 30 microg ethinyl-estradiol and 150 microg desogestrel. *Contraception* **51**: 3.

Gawel MJ, Rose FC (1982) Platelet function in migraineurs. *Adv Neurol* **33**: 237–42.

Gervil M, Ulrich V, Olesen J, Russell MB (1998) Screening for migraine in the general population: validation of a simple questionnaire. *Cephalalgia* **18**: 342–8.

Goadsby PJ (1997) Current concepts of the pathophysiology of migraine. *Neurol Clin* **15**: 28–9.

Guillebaud J (1983) The 150/30 formulation. Experience in the United Kingdom. *J Reprod Med* **28**(suppl 1): 66–70.

Hanington E, Jones RJ, Amess JAL (1982) Platelet aggregation in response to 5HT in migraine patients taking oral contraceptives. *Lancet* i: 967–8.

Headache Classification Committee of the IHS (1988) Classification and diagnostic criteria for headache disorders, cranial neuralgias and facial pain. *Cephalalgia* **8**(suppl 7): 1–96.

Heinemann LAJ, Lewis MA, Thorogood M et al. (1997) Case-control study of oral contraceptives and risk of thromboembolic stroke: results from international study on oral contraceptives and health of young women. *Br Med J* **315**: 1502–4.

Kalendovsky Z, Austin J, Steele P (1975) Increased platelet aggregability in young patients with stroke. *Arch Neurol* **32**: 13–20.

Kirowat O, Patanayindee A, Koetsawang S, Korver T, Bennink HJ (1998) A 4-year pilot study on the efficacy and safety of Implanon, a single-rod hormonal contraceptive implant, in healthy women in Thailand. *Eur J Cont Rep Health Care* **3**: 58–91.

Kittner SJ, Stern BJ, Feeser BR et al. (1996) Pregnancy and the risk of stroke. *New Engl J Med* **335**: 768–74.

Kubba A, Wilkinson C (1998) *Recommendations for Clinical Practice: Emergency Contraception.* London: Faculty of Family Planning and Reproductive Healthcare of the RCOG.

Lidegaard O (1993) Oral contraception and risk of a cerebral thromboembolic attack: results of a case-control study. *Br Med J* **306**: 956–63.

Lidegaard O (1995) Oral contraceptives, pregnancy and the risk of cerebral thromboembolism: the influence of diabetes, hypertension, migraine and previous thrombotic disease. *Br J Obstet Gynaec* **102**: 153–9.

MacGregor EA (1999a) *Managing Migraine in Primary Care.* Oxford: Blackwell.

MacGregor EA (1999b) *Migraine in Women.* London: Martin Dunitz.

MacGregor EA, Guillebaud J (1998) Recommendations for clinical practice. Combined oral contraceptives, migraine and ischaemic stroke. *Br J Fam Plan* **24**: 53–60.

Mazal S (1978) Migraine attacks and increased platelet aggregability induced by oral contraceptives. *Aus NZ J Med* **8**: 646–80.

Osterhaus JT, Townsend RJ, Gandenk B, Ware JE (1994) Measuring the functional status and well-being of patients with migraine headache. *Headache* **34**: 337–43.

Peatfield RC (1987) Can transient ischaemic attacks and classical migraine always be distinguished? *Headache* **27**: 240–3.

Rasmussen BK, Jensen R, Schroll M, Olesen J (1991) Epidemiology of headache in a general population — a prevalence study. *J Clin Epidemiol* **44**: 1147–57.

Russel MB, Olesen J (1996) A nosographic analysis of the migraine aura in a general population. *Brain* **119**: 355–61.

Salem HT, Salah M, Aly MY et al. (1988) Acceptability of injectable contraceptives in Assiut, Egypt. *Contraception* **38**: 697–710.

Samsioe G (1994) Coagulation and anticoagulation effects of contraceptive steroids. *Am J Obstet Gynecol* **170**: 1523–7.

Selby G, Lance JW (1960) Observations on 500 cases of migraine and allied vascular headache. *J Neurol Neurosurg Psychiat* **23**: 23–32.

Shearman RP (1964) *The Effect of Ovulation*

Inhibitors on the Ecretion of Urinary Steroids.
Searle Symposium. Sydney: GD Searle.

Slugg HJ, Lawson JP (1967) Side effects of oral contraceptives. *Lancet* **ii**: 612.

Somerville BW (1970) The use of continuous progestogen contraception in the treatment of migraine. *Med J Austr* **1**: 1043–5.

Somerville BW (1975) Estrogen-withdrawal migraine. *Neurology* **25**: 239–50.

Speroff L, Glass RH, Kase NG (1994) *Clinical Gynecologic Endocrinology and Infertility.* Baltimore: Williams & Wilkins.

Stewart WF, Schecter A, Rasmussen BK (1994) Migraine prevalence. A review of population-based studies. *Neurology* **44**(suppl 4): S17–S23.

Task Force on Postovulatory Methods of Fertility Regulation (1998) Randomised controlled trial of levonorgestrel versus the Yuzpe regimen of combined oral contraceptives for emergency contraception. *Lancet* **352**: 428–33.

Tzourio C, Iglésias S, Hubert JB et al. (1993) Migraine and risk of ischaemic stroke. *Br Med J* **307**: 289–92.

Tzourio C, Tehindrazanarivelo A, Iglésias S et al. (1995) Case-control of migraine and risk of ischaemic stroke in young women. *Br Med J* **310**: 830–3.

Wilkinson M, Williams K, Leyton M (1978) Observations on the treatment of an acute attack of migraine. *Res Clin Stud Headache* **6**: 141–6.

Wollersheim H, Pijls N, Thien T, van der Werf T (1987) Multiple vasospastic manifestations during ergot therapy. *Neth J Med* **30**: 75–9.

[WHO] World Health Organization Collaborative Study of Cardiovascular Disease and Steroid Hormone Contraception (1996a) Ischaemic stroke and combined oral contraceptives; results of an international, multicentre, case-control study. *Lancet* **348**: 498–505.

[WHO] World Health Organization (1996b) *Improving Access to Quality Care in family planning. Medical Eligibility Criteria for Initiating and Continuing use of Contraceptive Methods.* Geneva: WHO.

[WHO] World Health Organization Special Programme of Research, Development and Research Training in Human Reproduction; Task Force on Long-Acting Systemic Agents for the Regulation of Fertility (1978) Multinational comparative clinical evaluation of two long-acting injectable contraceptive steroids; norethisterone oenanthate and medroxyprogesterone acetate. 2. Bleeding patterns and side effects. *Contraception* **17**: 395–406.

WHO Collaborative Study of Cardiovascular Disease and Steroid Hormone Contraception (1998) Cardiovascular disease and use of oral and injectable progestogen-only contraceptives and combined injectable contraceptives. *Contraception* **57**: 315–24.

Couples with learning disabilities

Elaine Cooper

'Learning disability' is a blanket term which covers a
multitude of conditions and great variation in degree of
disability. It is usually described as 'a significant impairment
of intelligence and social functioning before adulthood', the
definition used by the NHS Executive Health Services for
People with Learning Disability. This definition is broad and
encompasses mild, moderate, severe and profound disability.
Individuals will often not fit precisely into these categories; it
is important always to see people with learning disabilities as
individuals, and to make a careful assessment of abilities, level
of comprehension, strengths and weaknesses in every case. It
is essential to remember also that all people with disabilities
are just that, people first who have a disability, and so have
hopes, desires, anxieties and problems like everyone else.

Couples with learning disabilities include couples where only
one partner has a disability, and those where partners may
have different degrees of disability. This affects the dynamics
of the relationship, and the views of the less able person can
be overlooked. As in all consultations concerning
contraception the viewpoint of both individuals is valid. In
some consultations the partner or carer may take over and

speak for the less able person. This can of course happen when neither partner has a disability!

Problems in obtaining contraception

Attitudes and assumptions

There are frequently barriers to overcome for people with disabilities when accessing contraception services. Some of these are due to assumptions and attitudes to such people when sexuality is involved. Many believe that learning-disabled people are not interested in sexual activity or that they will be unable to enter sexual relationships. A strong factor in this is the media—and thus society's—image of disability. This perceived image affects not only learning-disabled people themselves, but also their partner or potential partners, parents, professional carers and others such as health-care workers. Contraceptive services are thus deemed unnecessary. Others believe that such people will be very sexually active and indiscriminate in relationships, fostering the view that all people with learning disabilities require contraception to avoid multiple unplanned pregnancies. Both these views are offensive. Reality lies between these two extremes. Some people wish to be sexually active and thus contraception and safer sex are important as for all sexually active people.

It is important that professionals working with learning-disabled men and women recognize their own attitudes and assumptions to sexuality and disability and how it affects their working practice. They may interfere with effectiveness in identifying and meeting the clients' needs.

The attitudes and assumptions of health-care professionals may hamper their effectiveness in working with learning-disabled clients

Aside from these sociological, attitudinal problems, couples may fail to access services because they are unaware that contraception exists at all. The implications and consequences of being sexually active may not have been explained. Sometimes sex education has not been given or offered due to assumptions of non-activity, or has been delivered in a way that did not seem relevant at the time or was unintelligible. In addition, the couple may not have the ability to go unaided to a surgery or clinic. This may entail asking others, such as parents or carers, and this may not be acceptable to either party. Even if the couple are aware and can attend without assistance they may not have the words to ask for what they want, and indeed may be aphasic.

Problems with communication

If we consider the prerequisites for contraception methods in the population at large, the choice needs to be safe, non-intrusive and convenient, preferably separated from the time of sexual intercourse, effective, and suitable to the individual's lifestyle and preferences. All these criteria apply when a contraceptive method is being considered by and for a person or couple with a learning disability. Unfortunately, people with such a disability may find it difficult to recognize and verbalize these needs before being able to make an informed choice. In their everyday life they often experience other people influencing them and making decisions for them, with which they are expected to comply. This can apply to the need for or a choice of contraceptive method. It is incumbent upon the health professional, in the consultation, to ensure that clients are able to make their own choices. Sometimes an individual or couple may ask for their carer to be present to give them confidence. However, it can be helpful to see them alone for at least part of the consultation.

Learning disability may co-exist with physical disability, and the effect of this on the advisability and implementation of a particular contraceptive method needs consideration.

Cognitive and communication skills may be affected by the learning disability. Both of these aspects will influence whether a consultation is effective or not. Where understanding is impaired, it is essential to identify what the level of understanding is. To do this, some communication must be established. Clients who are aphasic may be able to understand what is said, but are unable to ask questions. In these cases communication may be aided by using Makaton (a form of sign language), or a Bliss board (with squares containing a symbol, letter or phrase) or a computer. The disabled person will be familiar with this mode but health professionals may find it daunting until they are familiar with it. Often the client is happy to initiate the professional in the ways of the chosen mode of communication. It is essential to establish a common language, regardless of its mechanism, for instance using words that the clients understand for parts of the body. As previously mentioned, sex education may have been neglected, not offered, or not understood. It may have been perceived as irrelevant by the user or the person teaching it. Using pictures to identify relevant words is helpful.

In all consultations it is essential to work at the pace of the less able partner

In all consultations with couples with learning disabilities it is essential to work at the pace of the less able partner. Unless the conversation is followed it will be difficult or impossible for a real choice to be made, and unless it is clearly understood how to implement a method there will be a high likelihood of contraceptive failure. Unless professionals are familiar with working with people with impaired understanding, they will need to be especially aware of adapting their pace to the couple's ability. Clients may need time to assimilate what has been said before they can formulate a response—they have to grapple with understanding what is said, finding suitable words to respond, and then enunciating them. In this context it is important to ask simple questions and not to raise several options in one question which may overwhelm the client, causing confusion and unreliable answers. Sometimes 'I don't know' can mean just that, or that the question is too difficult to answer. Sometimes irrelevant statements are made to divert away from the topic. These need to be acknowledged, but then the couple pulled back to the matter in hand.

Speech and language therapists may be able to help in cases of communication difficulties

When communication is a problem, help can be sought from speech and language therapists. They are often involved in therapy with people with learning disabilities and are skilled at aiding effective communication, and can often provide resources such as flash cards with symbols.

Many clients will attend the clinic or surgery, possibly with the help of a third party such as carer or parent. Some clients will find this too difficult and may need a home visit or visit at their day centre (e.g. by the domiciliary family planning service). Being on their own territory may give clients confidence, and as this increases they can be integrated into the clinic service or attend the general practitioner's surgery.

The issue of informed consent is crucial in dealing with vulnerable people

Legal aspects

It is important when working with people with learning disabilities to work within an ethical and legal framework (Carson 1987, Gunn 1991). These people are a very vulnerable group. The key issue is that of consent, which must be informed consent. When working with young people clinicians are familiar with the concept of 'Gillick competence': this allows young people under the age of 16 years to seek and obtain contraceptive services without parental consent, providing certain conditions are fulfilled. The most important of these conditions is an understanding of what is involved and the implications and consequences of contraception and sexual activity. Where there is a marked degree of learning disability this condition will not be fulfilled and the person will not be Gillick competent, so that parental involvement is necessary or that of the non-parent carer in some circumstances. When the young person reaches the age of majority then no one can answer for them and where major decisions are required (e.g. for permanent actions such as termination of pregnancy or sterilization) the courts need to be involved, i.e. legal opinion is necessary. In all consultations consent is important. This becomes vital where clinical examinations need to be undertaken as part of the consultation procedure. It is essential that the person knows who the clinician is and why the examination is being undertaken. This would be especially so in the management of an intrauterine device (IUD), cap or diaphragm, and for cervical screening, as vaginal examination is involved.

Choosing a method of contraception

When discussion of the various methods of contraception takes place, the available options are the same as for everyone else. No assumptions should be made and all options can be considered in light of the individual's preference, understanding and skills. For instance, a good memory is required to be an effective contraceptive pill-taker, to remember to insert a diaphragm or cap, or to use a male or female condom. A good memory is not required for an IUD, intrauterine system (IUS), implant or injectable contraception; but it must always be remembered that this group of long-acting methods do need checking and renewing at certain intervals or the method becomes ineffective (IUDs need changing, implants need replacing and further doses of injectable agents are required). The onus is on the provider to organize a recall system.

Assumptions are sometimes made that people with learning disabilities will be unable to manage oral contraceptive pill-taking satisfactorily. This may be so for some, but others, although probably needing reminding and supervision in the early days, may become effective and reliable pill-takers. Although it may take some time for a pattern of behaviour to be learnt, once learnt it may be unshakeable.

As always, effective and accurate teaching of the 'rules' for using a method of contraception is essential for reliable usage and low failure rate, and this is even more important when there is impairment of understanding. Visual reminders such as marking on a calendar can be helpful.

All the contraindications, absolute or relative, that apply to using a method of contraception will need to be considered, as in all contraceptive consultations.

Hormonal methods

If hormonal contraception is considered, both the formulation and route of administration need to be explored. Many people with learning disabilities take medication, commonly anticonvulsants for control of epilepsy. It is important to investigate which drugs are being taken and to find out whether there is a drug interaction; for example, if the anticonvulsant drug has a liver enzyme-inducing effect the dose of contraceptive pill will need to be increased to maintain effective contraception. Not all anticonvulsants are liver enzyme-inducing drugs. Each drug taken should be noted and data sheets and drug information services used if the situation is not clear. If a liver enzyme-inducing anticonvulsant such as carbamazepine (Tegretol) or phenytoin (Epanutin) is being used, a combined oral contraceptive pill containing 50 µg needs to be prescribed, not the usual 30 µg or 35 µg pills. In addition to a lack of effect at the lower doses there may be

an increase in breakthrough bleeding, which may lead to pill use being discontinued. To deal with this problem it may be necessary to prescribe doses of up to a maximum 90 µg in steps by adding pills together using combinations of 20, 30, 35 and 50 µg pills to make the total dose. This does not comply with current data sheets but is recognized clinical practice. The pill-free interval should be reduced to 4 days. Carbamazepine is sometimes prescribed for behavioural problems, not only for epilepsy. Similarly progestogen-only pills, of whichever formulation, would need to be taken in a higher dosage (two per day instead of one) and the time interval between injections of depot medroxyprogesterone acetate (Depo-Provera) or norethisterone oenanthate (Noristerat) reduced to 10 weeks and 6 weeks respectively.

Many people with learning disabilities take medication which may lead to problems of drug interaction

If there is an increase in thrombosis risk, for instance due to immobility or severe seizures (as in status epilepticus) or other conditions predisposing to thrombosis, then the combined oral contraceptive pill is contraindicated. When oestrogen is contraindicated there is a wide choice of route of delivery with progestogen-only methods. Reliable pill-taking is paramount with the progestogen-only pill because the time restrictions leave less room for error. Where memory or daily compliance with the pill regimen is a problem, a longer-acting method can be an advantage. Injectable contraception is reliable and effective, but some women cannot or will not tolerate injections—some are indeed needle-phobic so that each injection is a major trauma, stressful for the user and for the person giving the injection.

Where compliance is a problem the longer-acting contraceptive implant is worthy of consideration. However, the ability to lie still for the lengthy insertion and removal procedures may be a problem. Norplant, the only implant available until 1999, has six rods, but the newer Implanon consists of one rod preloaded in a sterile unit, making its insertion and removal a quicker procedure (Croxatto and Makarainon 1998).

Problems with the menstrual cycle

A useful side-effect of hormonal contraception is its ability to control the menstrual cycle (Cooper 1995). Many young women with learning disabilities are distressed by bleeding and are unable to cope with periods. Some will be frightened and distressed by this uncontrollable loss, especially if they have struggled to become continent. Even when there is double incontinence and pads are worn all the time, bleeding can cause distress and difficulty for the young women and their carer. Smearing may occur especially if masturbation occurs during the period. This can be particularly difficult for instance in the classroom or day centre.

A benefit of hormonal contraception is the ability to control the menstrual cycle

The combined pill, if not contraindicated, offers several regimens, ranging from smaller planned periods at the usual monthly interval, 'tricycling' (taking three packets one after the other without a break) giving less frequent bleeds, to continuous pill-taking which abolishes the cycle so that there is no blood loss. If breakthrough bleeding occurs a pill-free interval of 4 days (if an enzyme-inducing drug is being taken) or the usual 7 days is advised, after which the regimen of pill-taking can recommence. Although some women have bleeding problems with injectable progestogen, amenorrhoea is common and the longer the method is used the greater the expectation of amenorrhoea. The progestogen-only pill does not give this control, the cycle being rather more erratic. Women using implants may experience bleeding problems initially but amenorrhoea may develop later.

Another aspect of the menstrual cycle that can cause difficulty is premenstrual syndrome (PMS). Existing behavioural problems can be exacerbated at this time, making management difficult. Both the combined pill and injectable agents are useful in this context. If symptoms return in the last weeks before the injection is due the injection can be given an equivalent number of weeks early to combat this (Broome 1992). For those women whose epileptic seizures are increased premenstrually (status epilepticus sometimes occurring), abolishing the cycle and hence the seizures is of great value.

Intrauterine methods

The levonorgestrel-releasing IUS is a combination of a hormonal method and an intrauterine device, and is another route of delivery for progestogens. This progestogen-bearing system affects the endometrium, leading to smaller periods with eventual amenorrhoea. The difficulty for some women with learning disabilities is the insertion procedure: some are frightened of this intrusive experience and cannot comply. Others find it difficult to lie still, sometimes because of muscular spasms,

which makes insertion difficult and even hazardous, as it is essential that care is taken in placing the device correctly.

Intrauterine devices have the advantage of needing no memory to be effective, but an unfortunate side-effect is the heavier, possibly longer, periods which as mentioned above may not be well tolerated. Patients who have epileptic seizures may have a seizure during insertion, so the practitioner carrying out the procedure should be aware of this and prepare accordingly. Women who choose an IUD but are fearful of the insertion procedure may have the device inserted under general anaesthesia, but this has other aspects to be considered. Often, given time, the continuing doctor–client relationship enables the woman to permit examination for checking and for insertion or changing of the device

Barrier methods

Diaphragms and caps are not usually a method of first choice. Many women have been discouraged from touching themselves and find inserting the device distasteful (as they do using tampons). The intrusiveness distresses them. In addition, forward planning is essential for effective diaphragm use and this is often not a strong point of people with learning disabilities. However, there will be women who will persist, and learned behaviour patterns can be very reliable. Two heads are better than one, and the partner can be useful in reminding the woman or assisting her with insertion.

As for all sexually active couples the practice of safer sex is very important. Paramount in this is the use of condoms (male or female). Many non-disabled people find this a difficult issue to negotiate and this can be the more so for people with learning disability. However, knowing you should use a condom is of no value unless you know exactly how to use it. Many people (men and women) with learning disabilities carry a condom as they have been told that it is a good thing to do but cannot use it because the practical skills have been overlooked. Sometimes people have been taught on fingers, bananas, cucumbers or broom handles. This can be confusing as some people with learning disability are very literal in their understanding and cannot make the link to these objects representing the penis. Life-like models are available and are valuable for practice in an atmosphere free from emotional stress.

Natural methods

Natural methods of contraception are theoretically an option, but are not useful in practice. These methods require observational skills and the ability to follow complicated instructions carefully, otherwise the failure rate is high. These skills are not usually well developed in people with learning disabilities.

Sterilization

The ultimately reliable method of contraception is sterilization. It is not uncommon for clinicians to be asked about such operations for young, often adolescent clients of either sex, as it is seen as removing the great worry of pregnancy and its sequelae for the young woman and her partner. Sterilization would indeed, achieve this, but would have no effect on vulnerability, risk of infection, coping with periods or premenstrual syndrome. All of these aspects are important. Sterilization is a major decision for anyone, with or without a disability, as it must be considered to be permanent. There must be careful exploration and explanation of what is involved in the operation and its consequences must be clearly understood by the client—i.e. no baby, *ever*.

There can be many problems for people with learning disabilities who wish to have children and couples are often actively discouraged from so doing (Campion 1995). Careful discussion is necessary about what is involved in being a parent and what skills are required, not only with a small baby but as the child grows. Some couples will cope with the help of parentcraft teaching and ongoing support. Couples need to be aware that because the needs of the child are paramount they will be under observation. They could find their child taken into care if they prove unable to cope. This situation is very distressing and needs to be explored as a possibility before conception. As previously indicated, legal opinion may need to be sought prior to sterilization; this is definitely so if the person to be sterilized is unable to give informed consent.

Emergency contraception

It is important for all sexually active couples to be aware of the existence and availability of postcoital contraception. This information should be given particularly to all condom users, and people with learning disabilities, their partners and carers, should be included in this. The couple may need assistance from the carer to obtain it.

It is important to inform clients about the availability of emergency contraception

Although some health professionals and others find discussing and prescribing contraception for people with learning disabilities difficult, it should be remembered that unless this issue is addressed there may be a much more difficult situation of termination of pregnancy or concealed pregnancy arising.

Case histories

Case 1

Amy, aged 24 years, has a moderate learning disability subsequent to brain damage. She has a young man, Zac, whom she considers to be her boyfriend. He lives in a different town so she sees him sporadically. They are sexually active when they are together. Amy likes the company of men and is easily persuaded to have sex with them, which she enjoys, as she says, 'I like sex'.

Amy needs protection against pregnancy and sexually transmitted infections. Her brain damage affects her memory, making it difficult to stick to plans. All methods of contraception were discussed:

- oral contraception, although not contraindicated medically, could be difficult for Amy to achieve reliably

- injectable contraception or an implant is a possibility

- intrauterine methods are not a first choice as Amy is nulliparous and her lifestyle puts her at risk of pelvic infection

- diaphragm or cap methods are not acceptable to Amy and not a good option because of her memory deficit

- condoms would be advisable in the prevention of infection but 'the men don't like them' and often refuse to use them. Amy requires a contraceptive method that she has control of without being reliant on her partners. The female condom is unacceptable to her.

After full discussion Amy opted for injectable contraception. Because of her medication (carbamazepine), depot medroxyprogesterone acetate is given at 10-weekly intervals. When the injection is given, the date the next is due is calculated and entered on Amy's calendar. One week before it is due she receives a reminder letter.

Amy understands the need for condoms 'to stop catching an infection', and knows how to use them. She is being encouraged and supported in developing skills to insist the man uses them.

Case 2

Diana, aged 32, and Will, aged 37, have been going out together for five years. They are engaged and making plans for their marriage and home. Diana has a moderate learning disability and Will mild learning disability. They are very anxious to do 'everything right'. They would like a baby one day, 'but not yet' as they do not feel they could cope yet. The couple were both involved in the discussion on all contraceptive methods available. Diana would like to take 'the pill'. Some discussion of the best time to take it took place. Will was eager to do his part and would act as a reminder to Diana that the pill was taken. They liked the idea of ticking off on a chart when it was taken and the days without. They were thus able to use their combined skills to ensure reliable pill-taking.

References

Broome M (1992) Depo-Provera for PMT (letter). *Br J Fam Plan* **18**: 29.

Campion MJ (1995) *Who's Fit to Be a Parent?* Ch. 7. London: Routledge.

Carson D (ed) (1987) *The Law and the Sexuality of People with a Mental Handicap.* Southampton: University of Southampton.

Cooper E (1995) The needs of people with a disability. *Br J Fam Plan* **21**: 31–2.

Croxatto H, Makarainon L (1998) The pharmacodynamics and efficacy of Implanon: An overview of the data. *Contraception* 58(suppl): S91–7.

Gunn M (1991) *Sex and the Law*. London: Family Planning Association.

Couples whom nothing seems to suit

Linda Egdell

15

There is today a wide choice of effective contraceptive methods. Unlike other branches of clinical practice, where the optimal treatment is decided by the clinician after assessment and diagnosis, in family planning work it is the contraceptive users themselves who will choose their own method. The role of the practitioner lies not in determining the best method on behalf of the client but in presenting the advantages and disadvantages of the available options. Where there is illness or disability the choice may be limited to methods without serious contraindication or unacceptable difficulty in use, but for most young, healthy couples there will be no medical reason for limiting choice. The method that they will choose, and also use happily and consistently, will depend upon a range of factors. These will include personal preferences, the stage of their relationship, the patterns of their sexual lives, how reliable they wish their method to be, cultural and ethical considerations, and so on. Herein lies the skill, variety and fascination of working in the contraceptive field.

Some contraceptive dilemmas

Family planning practitioners will all have had experience of clients with no particular health problems who, in spite of being adamant that they do not want a pregnancy, reject every method of contraception presented to them. Each new suggestion is countered with reasons why it is unacceptable. A woman will explain that she has tried 'every pill on the market' and suffered side-effects with all of them, that the 'coil' caused 'infections' and had to be removed, that the injections made her fat, and that her partner 'cannot' (or will not) use condoms. She will express horror when shown female barriers, and sterilization of either partner seems too final. It may be tempting to lose patience, to argue the merits of already rejected ideas, to continue to change pill prescriptions again and again, to become didactic and make the choice for her, or simply to send her away with yet more leaflets which will not be read and condoms which will stay in the cupboard.

In truth most people do not really want to use contraception. Surely couples would prefer to enjoy their sexual lives without the inconvenience and distraction of appliances that need forethought, or pills which must be remembered and which feature in repeated health scares. No one enjoys embarrassing visits to the doctor, or painful procedures. There are disadvantages and potential side-effects associated with most current birth control methods, and far from enhancing a couple's romantic and sexual life, contraception can be intrusive and spoil the spontaneity of lovemaking. It is only the anxiety about unintended conception or the fear of acquiring infection that drives the couple, or more usually the woman, to the doctor, the clinic, the chemist or the supermarket.

Most people do not really want to use contraception, but accept it as a practical necessity

In championing the benefits of contraception, family planning enthusiasts can lose sight of this. Furthermore, we sometimes forget, as we welcome the latest technological advance, that the ideal contraceptive has yet to be invented and perhaps may never be. In trying to find something acceptable the cards are often stacked against even the most motivated and conscientious of couples. Contraceptive choice is limited to methods that all fail one or more of the 'ideal method' criteria (see box).

Many factors will play a part in the choice of method and in how reliably it is used. People

THE IDEAL CONTRACEPTIVE WOULD:

be 100% effective
carry no risk to health
be free from any side-effects
be independent of sexual intercourse or be fun to use
possibly have aphrodisiac properties
be equally effective if used after sex
be readily available and preferably free
require no planning or preparation
not involve memory
need no visit to a doctor or clinic
involve no medical examination or procedure whether painful or not
protect against sexually transmitted infections
be acceptable to all cultures and religious groups
be immediately reversible

will change methods according to their circumstances, with different partners and at various stages in their lives. Consistent use of their chosen method will be subject to a host of influences. Contraceptive users have the right to break the rules if and when they decide to, without fearing the disapprobation of their doctors or other providers. Are the condom mishaps cited by so many women when presenting for emergency contraception often actually attempts to earn the right to treatment without censure, whereas in fact precautions were not taken on that occasion? Lovemaking is often best when it is unplanned, spontaneous and abandoned. Risk-taking is not confined to sex. It is fun and it is universal. So much for 'family planning'!

The ideal contraceptive has yet to be invented, and perhaps may never be

With so little going for it, it is surprising that many couples cheerfully and successfully use contraception with reasonable consistency and with so little complaint. In the UK General Household Survey (Foster et al. 1993), nearly three-quarters of the women aged 16–49 years responding to questions on contraceptive use were currently practising birth control, or had been sterilized or had partners who had undergone a vasectomy. Of the remaining 29%, most had valid reasons for not using contraception, including being already pregnant, trying to conceive, or not having a sexual partner. Only 2% of the total sample admitted that they were not using contraception because they did not like it. Evidently most couples reluctantly accept contraception as a practical necessity.

However, some people can find nothing that appeals, they have tried then rejected everything, they may have had repeated pregnancies or several abortions yet continue to run risks, they return time and again for emergency methods and stop using any method within a very short time. Their contraceptive histories can induce confusion and despair in the hearts of their physicians, to whom they present a special challenge.

Diagnosing the problem

Finding time to listen to the real problems and formulating a structured approach to diagnosis can yield surprising results. Taking a careful history is a useful way to begin.

Taking a contraceptive history

In any family planning consultation an early review of the contraceptive methods that the person has used in the past can be very informative. What have they tried already, for how long did they persevere, and what were the reasons for stopping? Was their choice based on real consideration of the methods, or made just to please the doctor? What were their feelings about each method? Have they ever conceived while using contraception? What was the reaction of their partner to using contraception, and was he or she cooperative? Were they deterred by the reactions of friends or family members? How much has adverse media publicity affected their confidence? What information do they have about the methods they have used and what do they know of the alternatives? What do they believe about the dangers of using certain methods, and are they aware of any non-contraceptive health benefits?

Some relevant answers may be forthcoming if the questions are constructive and conducted in a spirit of exploration and information-sharing rather than condemnation. Individual methods all have their own particular problems, but solutions may be at hand.

Condoms may have been rejected because of previous mishaps. In the 1993 report by the UK Family Planning Research Network, 85% of a sample of nearly 3000 women clinic attenders said they had used condoms at some time (UKFPRN 1993). In this group of past or present condom users 40% had experienced splitting or the condom coming off on at least one occasion. One in three were thereby deterred from trusting the method again. A discussion about the technique of condom use may be helpful. Some people use oil-based lubrication which may weaken the rubber, or the condom may be too wide and thus slip off easily, or too narrow and prone to bursting. Again, a common complaint is that 'he won't use them', or that the condom is uncomfortable. A discussion about different shapes and sizes of condoms, or a change to non-latex material, may restore faith in the method.

Female barriers may not have been considered or even suggested. If the contraceptive provider holds the view that diaphragms are unreliable, messy and outdated, the potential user is unlikely to have the opportunity to discover otherwise. Some couples prefer not to use hormones and are happier with simple, less medically oriented methods.

Female barrier methods may not have been previously suggested

In the western world the combined oral contraceptive pill is the most widely used method, although some countries have yet to sanction its use for fear of encouraging promiscuity. The pill has some obvious advantages, being highly effective in trials, its use unrelated to the act of intercourse and under the control of the woman. It is small wonder that it has been hailed as one of the better inventions of the twentieth century. However, some women feel that they are expected and obliged to take this wonder drug, and some men assume that their partners are on it.

Many women will take the pill happily for several years, whilst others experience disagreeable side-effects. Even if a complaint of weight gain can be triumphantly refuted by the evidence of the weighing scales, the bloated sensation and tight waistband may be genuine. Nausea can be transient or relieved by change in hormone dosage, but the careful listener may discover that certain pills— notably the sugar-coated ones—can engender feelings of sickness at the time of swallowing. For some women, swallowing any tablet can be difficult. Other untoward symptoms such as withdrawal headache, mood swings, skin problems, changes in libido and so on may be enough to cause the woman to stop taking her pill. The International Working Group on Enhancing Patient Compliance and Oral Contraceptive Efficacy, in their consensus statement in 1993, quoted first-year discontinuation rates as high as 50–60% in some US studies (International Working Group 1993).

For many women the routine of pill-taking is not easy. Missed pills can lead at least to irregular bleeding, itself a disincentive to continuing, and more seriously a reduction in efficacy. The International Working Group cited Scottish evidence that only 28% of women followed the manufacturer's instructions correctly. The Group advocated that clinicians spend more time educating women about side-effects, teaching accurate pill taking and selecting pill formulations with the lowest possible risk of adverse symptoms. They also called for improved pill packaging and clearer instructions.

Perhaps the recommendation made by the Royal Pharmaceutical Society of Great Britain in 1997—which aimed to improve adherence to all medication regimens—that the term 'compliance' (denoting obedience or 'following the doctor's orders') should be replaced by 'concordance' (implying a shared responsibility between doctor and patient) is also relevant to the contraceptive pill (RPS 1997). Fostering a climate of cooperation between patient and prescriber and an uncritical approach to non-adherent behaviour could lead to an honest appraisal of the most helpful options.

Hormonal methods that do not rely on memory are sometimes the answer. A 3-monthly injection with the probability of amenorrhoea is welcomed by many. However, some women feel that periods are necessary, and others hate needles. The slow return to fertility after using injectables is not ideal and doubts remain about long-term effects on health. Many women return late for repeat injections and may then be made to wait for several months for their periods to resume so they can restart. In her paper on discontinuation rates in users of injectable depot medroxyprogesterone acetate (DMPA), Potter (1999) cites evidence that this contraceptive is effective for at least 16 weeks, calls for less caution in giving late injections, and makes suggestions about improving adherence to appointment dates.

The levonorgestrel intrauterine system (IUS) is rightly popular but pre-insertion counselling about early side-effects, including prolonged bleeding and other symptoms, is essential to improve continuation rates. Contraceptive subdermal implants are also an attractive idea and their insertion can be seen as less invasive and embarrassing than the IUS. However, public confidence was dented by media stories of difficult removals following insertion by inexperienced fitters, and the newer implants will need to have fewer problems with menstrual irregularity if they are to gain widespread acceptance.

Pre-insertion counselling about side-effects is essential to improve continuation rates for the levonorgestrel IUS

Intrauterine contraceptive devices (IUCDs), whether loaded with hormones or copper, offer effective long-term contraception and require no effort on the part of the woman, but many women are deterred by the fear of insertion fuelled by horror stories from friends. The experienced coil fitter will take great care to make the procedure as pain-free as possible. Application of a tenaculum to the cervical os in a conscious woman is not always 'just a little pinch', and local anaesthesia should always be considered. Continuation rates will depend on good counselling and follow-up. Some women will insist on the removal of their device after a short time and often for apparently trivial reasons. They may cite vague discomfort, but examination reveals no malplacement or tenderness. Closer enquiry may reveal that it is the thought of 'something being inside me' which is intolerable. Partners may share the same disquiet and no amount of trimming the threads 'because he can feel them' will alter the demands for removal. Showing a couple an actual device during counselling before fitting can be useful because the device is often thought to be much larger and more threatening than it actually is.

Fitting an intrauterine device may require local anaesthesia

This systematic appraisal of a couple's previous contraceptive experience, together with discussion about methods which they have not yet tried, may provide clues to the reasons why nothing seems suitable. Counselling and education can change perception and facilitate choice of an acceptable future alternative. However, for many couples the answer may not lie in the methods themselves but in other underlying problems.

Discovering the hidden problems

With time and careful listening it is often possible to find the real reason why contraception is so difficult. This may be related to current life events, the individual's background, beliefs, culture or aspirations, or problems in the relationship between the couple. The following are a few examples taken from the author's thirty years of experience in family planning work.

The nature of the relationship

If the relationship is one in which mutual trust care and respect are evident, and where communication is effective, a couple will make joint decisions about contraception. Some men who genuinely feel that they should take some responsibility will enquire about the availability of a male pill. Where there is anger and resentment and a couple cannot talk to one another, or if there is friction, discord or even violence, then contraception is less likely to be used reliably. Why should she swallow a pill every day when he apparently does not care? Women often complain, 'I have gone through having the children—it is his turn now.' Contraception is less well used not only at the beginning but also towards the end of relationships.

The quality of the sexual relationship

The sole aim of contraception is to enable people to enjoy a fulfilling sexual life without the fear of unintended pregnancy. So why do some clinicians find it so difficult to ask about sex during a family planning consultation? Sexual problems may manifest themselves through difficulties with contraception. Frequent requests for changes of pill or method may indicate that it is the sex rather than the birth control that is unsatisfactory. When lovemaking is difficult then contraception may be abandoned. Clinicians who venture into this aspect of people's lives need to be sensitive and tactful, should themselves feel at ease and unembarrassed, and should preferably have had relevant training.

Shame and guilt

Where an individual feels guilty about sex, procuring and using contraception might seem to be compounding the sin. Embarrassment about negotiating safer sex with one's partner or visiting the surgery for contraception is very common. Although we live in apparently liberated times, in most cultures there is not yet an open and relaxed attitude to sex. The continuing inadequacy of our school-based sex education, the prurience of the tabloid press, the widespread double standards and hypocrisy, the preoccupation with pornography, the silence of parents, the inactivity of governments, the reluctance to allow contraceptive advertisements, and even the continuing poor image of condoms, all conspire to make sex a guilty secret and contraception a taboo subject.

Furthermore, for some people their personal experience, the culture of their families or their religious upbringing may bring particular problems. In exploring patients' feelings and history one needs to be prepared to deal with disclosures of previous abuse.

Preoccupation with other problems

Finding the inclination, time or energy to organize contraception can be difficult in the face of other more immediate and pressing problems and it is always worth looking at the couple's circumstances. Are there financial worries or housing problems? Unemployment may be an issue or there can be work-related stresses. Perhaps there are concerns relating to the children or to elderly relatives. Family life may be chaotic, or the neighbours a threat. There may be no instant solutions, but talking may help.

Fatalism

Contraception represents power. It is enabling. It allows couples to delay having a family in order to finish education, establish a career, amass material wealth, or travel around the world. It lets people decide not only when but whether to have children. Contraception permits spacing between pregnancies and an end to reproducing. However, for some people the belief that they have the ability to direct the course of their lives, to influence events or to change things is alien. The feeling that what will be will be, the fascination with horoscopes, the meek acceptance of whatever life throws at one, can counteract the motivation to take any steps oneself.

Ambivalence

Is there an underlying and unacknowledged desire for pregnancy? A woman who has recently undergone a therapeutic abortion will sometimes show a surprising lack of consistency in using contraception during the ensuing weeks and months. This may be an unconscious attempt to come to terms with her decision to terminate. It may also be true that some couples value the possibility of pregnancy even if it is not really wanted. Perhaps there can be too much 'family planning'! Other women may really want the reassurance that they could become pregnant if they wanted to. Now that childbearing is being delayed, women do worry that they might in the event be infertile. For a man a pregnancy can be proof of his virility.

Depression and poor personal esteem

Sadly, some women do not feel worthy enough to care about looking after themselves. Hidden emotional or mental health problems can affect all areas of a person's life.

When nothing at all is suitable

It has to be said that there are still some couples who, although highly motivated to use contraception and without any particular problems, nevertheless have very real difficulty in finding a suitable method. This is hardly surprising given the imperfections of most of the currently available contraceptives. Until the ideal contraceptive is launched the choice of what to use is all too often a compromise, but assisting men and women in their decisions can be rewarding. Much of the fascination of family planning practice is in listening to people, learning about their lives, observing their relationships, sharing in their happiness and disappointments, enjoying their humour and sometimes, but not often, knowing that one may actually have helped.

Case histories

Case 1

Jane is 43 years old and attends for emergency contraception because a condom split. She has four children ranging in age from 5 to 15 years. Her combined pill was discontinued because of her blood pressure. An IUCD was removed because of heavy bleeding, and DMPA injections caused severe mood changes. She has conceived in the past while using a cap. 'I don't seem to have much luck with contraception,' she complains. A friend had side-effects with a levonorgestrel intrauterine system. Jane herself does not want any more hormones and she is frightened of general anaesthesia. Her new partner refuses vasectomy because he has no children of his own. The only solution seems to be abstinence or careful condom use.

Case 2

Olwen is only 16 years old. She first came to the clinic with her mother when she was 14 because she was having unprotected sex. A combined pill was prescribed. During the next year she attended several times because of breakthrough bleeding and other side-effects. Careful questioning uncovered her erratic pill-taking and poor recall of how to take it. She found it very difficult to remember, and her mother was having problems of her own and was not supportive. 'She's a stupid girl,' her mother says. She was terrified of injections, so pill-taking was re-taught on numerous occasions. She finally gave it up and became pregnant.

After the baby was born she was given the pill again when she had her postnatal check at the surgery. Following further breakthrough bleeding she abandoned the pill and conceived again when the baby was 5 months old. Following termination of this pregnancy she was given a DMPA injection. This caused prolonged bleeding so she did not return for a second injection. She reappeared at the clinic for emergency contraception. Future contraception was discussed but she was adamant that she did not want an IUCD, and her boyfriend would not use condoms although they definitely did not want another pregnancy.

Life is very difficult for Olwen. She and her boyfriend are living in a council flat on a depressed estate. She tries hard with the baby and is proud of her flat. They have little money and her boyfriend is about to lose his job. Now the neighbours have started causing trouble. Her family seems to have forgotten about her. Contraception is the least of her problems.

The only hope for Olwen would appear to be to somehow reassure her that an IUCD would significantly improve her life.

References

Foster K, Jackson B, Thomas M, Hunter P, Bennett N (1993) *General Household Survey. OPCS Social Services Division.* London: Government Statistical Service.

International Working Group (1993) A consensus statement: enhancing patient compliance and oral contraceptive efficacy. *Br J Fam Plan* **18**: 126–9.

Potter L (1999) Why must one 'restart' a method that is still working? A case for redefining injectable discontinuation. *Fam Plan Perspect* **31**(2): 98–100.

[RPS] Royal Pharmaceutical Society of Great Britain (1997) *From Compliance to Concordance: Towards Shared Goals in Medicine Taking.* London: RPS.

[UKFPRN] UK Family Planning Research Network (1993) Mishaps occurring during condom use, and the subsequent use of post-coital contraception. *Br J Fam Plan* **19**: 218–20.

Index